To Debbie

God bless the caregivers!

Rose M. Grant

I LEFT MY MEMORY ON A BUS SOMEWHERE

A Bittersweet Journey through Alzheimer's Disease

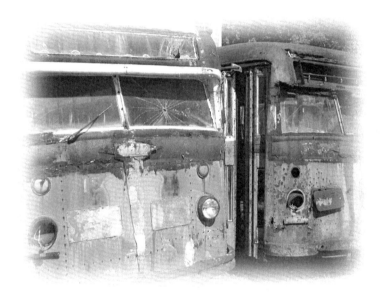

Rose M. Grant

———◦•‡•◦———

Dedication

This remembrance is dedicated, of course,
to my husband Jack
and our two wonderful children,
Kevin and Heather

———◦•‡•◦———

In Gratitude

I would like to thank the following people who provided free, compassionate, dependable day care for Jack for six months: Brian Grant, Kevin Grant, Don Carroll, James T. Crofton, the late William Golden, Carol A. Mello and Charlene Orton. I could not have made it through those last months without you. I will always be grateful for your friendship and generosity.

Thank you to the biggest and best support group anyone could ever have--the Bishop Stang High School family. Your physical and spiritual support continues to keep me afloat.

Thank you to all of the professionals who took such good care of Jack and me over the years: Ehab Sorial, M.D., Paulette M. Masse, M.S., L.S.W., Jim Sullivan, L.S.W. and the staff at Southcoast Health, Charlton Memorial Hospital, Fall River, MA.

A very special thank you is given to Dr. Duane Bishop who had the very difficult task of telling us Jack's diagnosis and who encouraged me to write this book.

Gratitude is sent to the staff and my coffee club friends at New Boston Bakery for giving me ears to listen and shoulders to cry on. You saved me many hours of therapy. Remind me to buy you a cookie.

I extend my deep appreciation to the staff at Country Gardens Nursing Home who not only did the challenging job of providing daily care to Jack, but who became his second loving family.

Finally, thanks go to James Pavao, whose support and encouragement spurred me on to see this project to completion.

Rose M. Grant

As I was walking up the stair

I met a man who was not there

He was not there again today

Oh, how I wish he'd go away.

OLD ENGLISH NURSERY RHYME

———◆◆◆———

God never gives us more than we can handle.

I just wish he would not trust me so much.

MOTHER TERESA

CHAPTER ONE

The Disease

By the time you read to the bottom of this page, at least one new diagnosis of Alzheimer's disease will have been made. And chances are good that you will know that person or at least their loved one. This is because a new patient is added to this dubious rank every sixty-eight seconds.

Currently, Alzheimer's disease ranks sixth in the cause of death for Americans and is one of the only diseases where you will never see a celebration of survivors. Treatments and survival rates for most kinds of cancer and HIV continue to improve but progress for Alzheimer's treatment has been painfully slow for those five million families dealing with this terrible theft of a family member.

The average time span from diagnosis to death is ten years. This is a long time to provide care, to tax the health care system and to watch a loved one slowly leave this planet. While the late President Ronald Reagan's wife Nancy may not have been the first to use the phrase "a long goodbye," she is certainly the one to make it famous. Sadly, how well put.

This devastating disease is an expensive one. In 2014, the cost to our nation was $203 billion and it is estimated by the Alzheimer's Association that the bill will increase to $1.2 trillion by 2050. Considering that most caregivers (up to 15 million) are unpaid family members providing 17 billion hours of care, the financial burden is even more staggering. (Alzheimer's Association Fact Sheet, 2014)

Alzheimer's disease can be broken down into three phases of progression, aptly named Stages I (mild), II (moderate) and III (severe). During Stage I, the initial symptoms include the well-known short term memory loss, with difficulty concentrating, finding words, and making decisions. The patient is aware that something is wrong and at times becomes quite anxious about it. At others times, he seems quite himself and can cope with every day living. However, toward the end of this two to four year period, autonomy is slowly eroding away and the person becomes more and more dependent on his caregiver.

During Stage II, which can last anywhere from two to ten years, the disease becomes more obvious. Forgetting names, faces, words, and routines are all part of a normal day. This increases anxiety, which leads to suspiciousness, irritability, hallucinations, and sun-downing – all of which present greater challenges to the caregiver as their parent or spouse becomes angry, belligerent and unrecognizable as the lovable, intelligent, funny person he once was.

Stage III, also called the terminal phase, can range from several years to only a few months. During this time, the family member is totally unable to care for himself, which includes feeding, ambulating, hygiene, toileting and all of the rest of the activities we all take for granted in our two and three year old toddlers. Just as our loved one can no longer talk or walk, they also begin to have serious swallowing problems and this loss becomes the beginning of the end.

In the spring of 1995, my husband Jack and I began our long goodbye.

CHAPTER TWO

Our Story

———

March 1, 1998

My husband and I met at Bishop Stang High School in September of 1971. I was a rookie biology teacher and he was the guru art teacher across the hall. All of the kids hung out in "Bud's" room. He was the COOL teacher in the building. For the first two years we were just friends and colleagues, but a fateful school ski trip to Switzerland in February of 1973 brought us together, and four months later we were married. Despite (or because of) our thirteen year age difference, we were great pals and did all kinds of things together including camping, hiking, kayaking, and especially walking. We both loved the snow and the beach, so we always found something to do together. Together was the operative word.

Our son Kevin was born in November of 1975 and our daughter Heather followed a little over three years later, in January of 1979. During those years I left teaching to stay home with the kids, but managed to earn an MS in biology from the University of Massachusetts (Dartmouth). Jack already had an MFA in commercial design from Boston University. We always joked that we were a merger of the Arts & Sciences.

Jack had an on again-off again employment history due to the fact that art teachers were always the first to go whenever school systems had budget problems. So when I had a chance to teach part-time at Fisher College and Bristol Community College, I grabbed the positions. For one three year period I was the only one working while Jack was "Mr. Mom." Finally, in 1986, Jack was appointed to the faculty at Case Junior High School (after three years of unemployment and two years of working as a mental health aide). He was finally back teaching art and was happy. Coincidentally, I was offered my old position at Stang, so we both went back to teaching full time that fall. Things were good.

After a few years, Jack started having some physical problems- upset stomach, diarrhea, noisy bowels, insomnia. These symptoms would always begin to appear around October, force him to the doctor by November, and disappear after school got out in June. Antacids, anti-diarrheal meds and various anti-depressants became part of our lives. Because middle school students are often a challenge, we thought these symptoms were stress related. Then other things started happening. Jack began losing things all the time, like his Swiss Army pocketknife, glasses, keys, grade book. Complaints were being made about Jack's performance at work. His principal said he needed to alter his curriculum and mentioned that he was missing paperwork deadlines and meetings. Again, we blamed these things on stress and the fact that he was never very organized anyway. But the pressure from the administration escalated and Jack filed a grievance with the teachers' union, feeling that he was being harassed. Back we went to the doctor's office with more complaints and for more tests. Finally, we were given a referral to a psychiatrist for treatment for depression. The psychiatrist noticed Jack's forgetfulness and ordered a complete neurological work-up. An electroencephalogram and CAT scan both returned normal but other tests showed significant problems with short-term memory. A more comprehensive memory assessment was scheduled at Rhode Island Hospital and the diagnosis was "amnestic syndrome." No one was saying Alzheimer's disease but we all were thinking it. The doctors at

Rhode Island Hospital, as well as our primary care physician and our psychiatrist, said that Jack had to quit working. In fact, they could not understand how he had managed to get through the days for as long as he did. The stress he had been experiencing was due to him trying to cope when he couldn't remember kids' names, which class he had next, what lesson he did yesterday, where he put his grade book, and so on. He had pulled it off by doing the same thing every day, every class. No wonder the students were giving him a bad time. They were bored. Kids that age are very perceptive. They probably knew something was wrong long before any of the doctors or other adults recognized it.

So, in the spring of 1995, after thirty years of teaching, Mr. Grant "retired."

CHAPTER THREE

Jack's Journal

Have you ever met couples who say they never argue? That actually was pretty much true with us. I am not saying that we always agreed with each other but Jack was pretty easy going and we would talk and work things out. As the Alzheimer's progressed, however, he often got upset with me for "making all of the decisions" for both of us. That wasn't true, but he could not remember discussing where we would go for Thanksgiving that year or what we would buy his mother for her birthday. So our doctor suggested keeping a "Teflon" journal. It was his amusing way of saying "nothing sticks," so write it down. We began making contracts for all kinds of events, from simple things such as a dentist appointment to going on a trip. I would type up all of the details and we would both sign and date it. When the time came to head out the door and he resisted, I would bring out the journal and show him the contract.

Later, he became very frustrated with keeping track of his reading and used his journal for that as well. It wasn't until a few years ago, reading his journal entries again, that I realized that his repetition of walking routes might also have been a coping mechanism he used for doing his beloved "traipsing" without getting lost.

Jack kept his journal on little pieces of paper. He resisted writing in a bound book, but later I got him to do so. Jack's journal entries have not been edited with the possible exception of name changes where necessary. The spelling and syntax are his.

November, 1998

November 23

Read Durant -Volume IV- The Age of Faith pp.614-649

Walk-Weetamoe to Ray to Valentine to Madison to Weetamoe to Greenlawn. A run later-a good run. Not in the best condition. Legs good. Breath no. Beautiful day, bright and cool.

November 24

Walk up weetamoe to Ray Street to Valentine to Elsbree to coffee & muffin. Home by President Ave and right on Highland. Another special day-bright and cool. Morning sky bright red- red cloud display. Rake leaves front & back. Good work. Yard developing slowly. Reed History Durant The Recovery of Europe 1095-1300.

Met Don Carroll & wife after coffee. Looks great (of course). Met on way from the pastry shop on New Boston Rd. We generally walk over for coffee and cookie (fresh made). A nice event each day when Rose gets home. Accoustics not good but we got used to it.

November 25

Heather is home from school. Doing very well in all departments. Presents positive affect across the board. She borrowed a car from a friend at school. Walked with Rose (Heather slept). Another great day. Bright sun and cool air. We went at a good pace.

Earlier on spent time and efford raking leaves.

Fireplace at work. Do not have the best technique and the wood is probably not the best but I think it is fine (I think that Rose feels the same).

November 26 - Thanksgiving

Fill five barrels with leaves stuffed in. Could fill another five barrels. I enjoy the ritual. I have always been a walk thru the autumn leaves type. Especially if windy and overcast. Walked with Rose -splended day for it.
Football 12:30 Pittsburg at Detroit. Watched game in Swansey. I sat next to Charly (father-in-law). He is in good condition but a bit weak. Met the people at Bark St. Memoraries regenerated. Very aware of the passage of time. Wins & losses. Approprialy it was a nice visit.

Heather is doing all of it correctly. Kevin is in the chapter titled "win some, lose some, go after each day". Reminds me of 1958.

All the players are in the game, each playing according to their circumstances. As all days, today was fine.

November 27

Morning walk with Rose. Great day clear with glareless sun, cool with lively breesy.

Heather home. She is doing well and makes me feel fine. Mom over and glad to sees Heathers. She's had a long life and is understandly proud of her kids and grandkids. There is a certain dignity that goes with a long, sometimes difficult life. Mom has a lot of pride and she shows it. God Bless Her.

Rose and Heather went out shopping. With abit of cabin fever, I took one of my walks. Down Weetamoe, around the block, and back up Weetamoe (very steep and a great workout). The landscape color in the sky, land and river, the wind in from the west all make a tirifical tour. With this is the physical workout that is regenerating. Thank Falls River for the hills that add so much to a mere traipse.

November 28

Started day with bagels and coffee. Followard with grocery shopping. Usually activity. The bagel shop is interesting. The bagel and cream cheese is very good (double toast the bagel!). Shaw's is bright, clean and well stocked. It's a great stop and watching Rose shop is impressive. I allways think of the A&P back in 1957, '58, '59. They were great days. Got the GI Bill stipend for school and worked part-time for the A & P. Played a million games of basketball, drank a million beers. Everyday was a celebration. Back then there were a number of good bars. I felt like the Student Prince. Usually we do some stuff around the house-today I put the lights on the pair of trees on the front lawn. One of our rituals. !look fore to it. Forego reading when others here. When I read I need quiet. Back to book tomorrow or Monday.

November 29

Another beautiful day. Bright cool breeze and clouds floating by. Rose & I took our walk with the usual pleasure. Walking is great for us and we can afford it! Heather went back to school. She presents as in control of a well directed life. God bless her.

Patriots win on the last play of the game- a pass with 1 sec. to go.

Rose is wrapping Christmas gifts. She always plans ahead and gets the necessary stuff done.

At this time, 8:18, the trees that have been decorated with lights look terriffic. They are somewhat thicker which meens we will have to add more lights.

Impossible to read the last couple of days. Looking forward to reading Durant's History. I read for I have always been a history nut.

Rose brought up the idea of going to Florida to visit Ernie & wife. Interesting. Glitz caused Heather to be late to school. We worried. Now OK.

November 30

Had looked forward to today as wen I would read History (Durant). Took a walk at 8:00 to coffee & muffin. Had plans to run in the pm. Things, however, needed doing in the yard. Also in the house. Vacuuming, etc. Of all places, the Marine Corps was the place that clean and neat was the way to go. Our (Rose & me) walking when I got a severe pain in the lower backside location. I was in bad pain. Walked home alone. (Rose finished her planned walk).

When I got home there were things that needed doing. So I did them. This sad story means that a) I had a terriffic rectal pain and b) I was compelled to do some stuff around the house that I had postponed and c) the third plague was that I could not read today. (History of course) I am on page 678 and am going to pg 1086 (The Age of Faith) Vol. 4. After this, 7 more volums. And I am a day dreamer. Won't be done soon!

December, 1998

December 1

More polite weather. Mild, light breeze, heavy overhead clouds. To west it cleared until past Swanseay.

Just another seene on a traipse. The most important aspect of a walk is the eyes.

(Still reading Durant- topics and page numbers from 678-702 listed. The following journal entry refers to this reading.)

There is so much information in "The Age of Faith" the read-inds can be overpowering in the sheer amount of information. Many of the names and places and events are all memoies from when I taught world history at Stang (along with art and mechanical drawing along with driving the bus to the games). Reading this demands concentration and I have to focus more than a few times in or der to insure my understandance. I look forward to tomorrows reading (also the walk).

December 2

Morning walk. Good walk at brisk pace. Bright sky with cloud apostrophes. A nice route, low trafic, clean streets & well kept homes (the Highlands!). Later down weetamoe to Mian around the block & back up Weetamoe. Terriffic workout & scenery. I hope no one catches it. I'm selfish when it comes to traipsing about.

December 3

Have not run in some time. Decided to go today. I did better than I thought I would.

I walked the small hill of the water reservoir. Feel great for performance. Looking forward to more running.

Rose at school late 6:30. She is involved with lots of activities. She is the ideal teacher.

December 4

I can still feel yesterday's run. Down Weetamoe, etc. I enjoy the idea that I got back to running. Today I factored in my age and condotion and decided to persue this endevor carefully. Later, a traipse to the barber. A good guy-plenty of tattoos and no talk. He will to bikers, tho. Back home - another corking day. Begin reading history.

December 5

Another beauty Sunday. Holy Name Church always presents the reserved architecture that prevents a mjor jump from that which is our daily life and that which is the messaric and metaphisic program of the Roman Catholic Church. We had the Irish priest who tends to go on verbally. I have to admit that I cannot understand a lot but I am away of the Irish interpenert of the big mission. This stays anyone who has gone to mass every Sunday since 1940. The message is the right one and it gives major meaning to life.

After reading the Fall River and then the Providence papers, I have no energy to read anymore. The wandering Patriots won a big game against the Pittsburg Steelers. A great game to watch. I feel, however, that soccer (Europe futbol) is superior to the American product. Mass assault with uniforms!

The Christmas season lights are now alight. The message is still there- 2000 years of the right stuff.

Rose and I took an afternoon walk and as usual it was as is all of our traips- in many ways just an other event. I think it is quite special. I know Rose feels the same. Lucky Jack, Lucky Ro.

December 6 & 7

The great weather continues. It can never bore The weather commands a good quick march about the city. Droped down Weetamoe (great work for the knees & thighs going down-all the way up is great for heart, lungs, legs). A great hill which also presents great views of Somerset, clouds, trees, yards and the microgardens growing in the gutters, between the curbs and the cement. A feast of backyards never tires the eye, which never tires of verity!
Have done yard work each day. Some days just picking and replacing. The yard is slowly going to a very pleasant yard. It will never get there. The important thing is to get toward there! I under stand why the ancients placed gardens and yards as domicel to the Gods.

December 9

Rose & I went to the coffee shop on New Boston Road. A nice ritual. A walk with chit chat. A small view of a place that is just right. Well made homes, well kept, various displays of the unity of well designed sites and pleasant homes. Good Fall River. This walk is always good.

Mel just came in at 9:28 PM. Good cat!

Catching into efficiently reading. Formally a careless but now more of a careful reader.

December 10

No major walk today. Will go for coffee and cookie when Roro gets home. A pleasant stop with bad accoustics.

Life is like that. Some times a good set up is not what it could be. This is one of my proofs that life is not perfect. It is great fun but it is not perfect. Fortunally the talk there is mostly banter. Of course this is the view of an old crab (me). That's part of the fun. I don't have to be serious. Great read today. The more I read "The Age of Faith", the more I want! The Lucky Guy!

December 12

Got Christmas tree and installed in the great room. The base diameter is about the same as the higtht. This robust tree should be a sight indeed!

December 13

No read today. Day to take care of house cleaning. Some small yard work-trim the holly in front- trying to have vertical as apposed to wise spread character. Great deal of work in cleaning hose. The tree just standing there wateing for its decorations. Perhaps tomorrow. Footbal good. No good (not worth a ---!).

December 14

Today's walk up Weetamoe & northbound on Ray. Cool Breezey with bright sun. Could be called a perfect day. 1'1' call it that. This autumn has been outstanding in the weather department. Right on Valentine & South on Elsbree to Langley. Right on President to Ray south bound down by Hood & and by the school (the kids all running and running and running) and down to McDonald's for coffe and a bran muffin. The Brilliant sky improves everything. The nice thing is that there is no charge for it. Thanks, God. Back home by President to

Robeson and by the school there. The kids here are doing what they are supposed to do (run an chase each other). It reminds me of the school yard at my school- Sacred Heart 1940-1949. I wore out the knees of lots of knickers. When someone was chasing me (tag) I had a trick to ad void being tagged. I would drop to one knee (from a full speed run). Many times I missed to tag but I put holes in all my knickers. The shoes (no sneakers here) took a good beating.

After coffee I decidede to drop down Weetamoe, circle the old St. Josephs school and bye our house in 1949 (next to the cemetary North End). Lots of memories here.

Reading	Chapter
The Resurrection of the Arts	XXXI 1095-1300
I. The Esthetic Awakening	pp 845-847
II. The Adornment of Life	847-851
III. Painting	
1. Mosaic	851-852
2. Miniatures	852-853
3. Murals	853-856
4. Stained glass	856-857
IV. Sculpture	857-862
The Gothic Flowering	XXXII 1095-1300
I.The Cathedral	pp. 863-868
II. Ccntinental Romanesque 1066-1200	868-870
III. The Norman Style in England	870-872
IV. The Evolution of Gothic 1133-1300	872-875
V. French Gothic	875-882
VI. English Gothic	882-885
VII. German Gothic 1220-1300	885-887
VIII. Italian Gothic	887-890
IX. Spanish Gothic	890-893
X. Considerations	893-894

December 15

Start the day off with a brisk walk to Robeson & haed south. Go as far as Locust, follow it to Oak Grove and New Boston Road to Robeson and home. Check up on house and head out again. Up Weetamoe to Ray to Langly & take a right on Langly to Elsbree to the bagel shop for a mediam coffee and a world class bran mufee. It was gigantic and delicious. Having completed the feast I headed home up President Ave to Hood and down to Greenlawn.

Checked out the cat, house, garage and yard. All things copascetic, I walked doen Weetamoe, right on North main past the North Buryall grounds and left on the comer. Down Brightman to just before the bridge. Back on Brightman towards North Main, right to Weetamoe, up the hill. What a workout. The heart is working overtime all the way up. This is a great work out for the whole body. I try to do it as much as I can. Back at home I fix the outside lights on the front lawn trees-yes, again! The weather was perfect: cool & bright with occasional clouds. Later Rose & I drove to the coffee shop. Read.

December 16

(ROSE'S NOTE: not sure this date is accurate because I gave Jack his membership to the Boys' Club for Christmas. He cried like a baby when he opened the gift and realized what it was. This had everyone in tears. I suspect he actually wrote this journal entry some time between Christmas and the New Year.)

Continue roaming (actually at a quick march) the streets and hills of Fall River. Mostly in the North Highlands with forays into Somerset, Downtown, old neighborhoods-Linden St, Turner Park (Danfourth St, etc, etc, etc). I don't tire of revisiting the same places. There is a new rememberance or point of view. Things change.

A significant addition. Retounned to Boys Club on Bedford St. Brian takes down & back. Great work outs. Some of the guys from the 60s, 70s, 80s and new kids. I was somewhat worried as how it would be. I wasn't sure of this move.

January 1999

January 5

No excuse for reports on walking adventures. Human frailty! Walk every day. Best in cold, bight, breezy conditions. Rest assured that I have my daily regina.

January 6

Workout at Boys Club turned out to be very good. Brother Brian drive. Things seem good.

1. Fairly good condition
2. Access to all facilities-great workout
3. See some people from 10 years ago. A lot of the guys are still there from the old days.

Good workout. Good comradite stuff. I'm smiling. Many of the guys are HEAVY.

January 7

Shovelled snow on the beautiful day. Bright sun 28°. Walked down for a muffin at McDonald's, avoiding slush & snow (shoes).

Resume reading is like meeting an old friend.

Our usual walk to New Boston Road & coffee & cookey. I look to it (with Rose) each day. Tomorrow- Boys' Club 7:30 am and then Thomas Acquinas.

January 8

The Adventure of Reason
V. Thomas Aquinas 961-967
VI. The Thonist Philosophy

1. Logic	967 -968
2. Metaphysics	968-969
3. Theology	969-970
4. Psychology	970-972
5. Ethics	972-974
6. Politics	974-976
7. Religion	976-977
8. The Reception of Thomism	977-978
VII. The Successors	979-983

Reading Thomas Aquinas while the snow falls!!!

Have rejoined the Boys' Club. Brother Brian (one of the good guys) picks me up on MWF at 7:30 Good workouts.

January 10

No Historical reading (sold out to TV). Getting ready for our trip to Florida (!).

January 11

Good workout at Boys Club. Have been going MWF for a few weeks. Brian picks me up (which is a great situation). Basel workout-sit ups, push ups. Basktball workout. Today I strained a muscle in left leg on my 35th full court, full speed brakeaway lay up (this is a solo program-there are no defence problemes. Just open sprints.) I hope its not serious. An old guy (my age) said, "You're not twenty-one anymore." I said, "Twenty-one times three." Just then I got the message in the back of my left leg.

(Rose's note: Entries for 1-12 through 1-14 all pages from Durant's The Age of Faith)

January 20

For some reason, of which I have no idea, there early along I sensed a relation between reading and walking the streets and hills of Fall River, Tiverton and Somerset.

The daily walk and read has been a great adventure. J.P.G.

(Rose's note: Jack's journal entries at this point became sporadic and all are notations about reading from Durant's Age of Civilization. All of Jack's journaling was done on pieces of 4" X 6" white paper (his choice). He seemed to be having trouble keeping his writing going at this point, so I bought a journal that suggested what to write about, such as: "The weather today is... In the news today ")

April 24, 1999

The weather today is sunny and cool. Very light wind. A beautiful day.

Great sorrow today concerning the high school students who killed so many.

Rose is very busy with the drama presently at Stang. The kids are really enthusiastic and so is Rose. Very impressive! Each day I try to read 25 pages of world history- The Story of Civilization.

I feel very well. Each day I take a good walk. Typical-down Weetamoe over the bridge to Somerset. Now there is consideral work going on. The Brightman Bridge is to be replaced.

When I walk or read history I enjoy. Enclude yard work. Things that brighten my day are Rose, Kevin, Heather, Mel (the cat). When I cross trails with someone I've met before.

April 25 - Sunday - 10:28 AM

Another splendid day! Warn sun with mild cool breezes. In the news today- the damned business in Kosovo. According to Durant it has been going on since 13th cent.

Kevin at work at country club and Heather at Mount Holyoke doing well. Heather works hard and loves it. Same with Rose.

I am concerned about memory problems. It may be because I am not a good listener. Also I am a long time day dreamer (Poetic?). I am concerned about the changes that come with the passage of the years. Physically I fee! great. Mentally the issue is in doubt. Shakey memory!!!

There is no end to weeding the gardens-lawn. Every square inch has some interest. Every sky has interest-so on. There is always something to do.
Continue to read history at 25 pages per day. Sometimes I have difficulty staying with it. I come back to it.

We usually go to 10:00 AM mass. It is always the same and always different. We (me & Rose) have taken the same seat at mass. Rose tells me for 23 years. For some reason I don't sing during mass. I think of the days of the Latin masses and the

Latin mystery mass early in Sacred Heart Church. We lived next to the Sacred Heart School. We had a terrific school yard. We (the boys) played games in which one kid had to be caught or excape. It cost a lot in pants knees because of the tricky maneuvors to avoid being caught. We sum war knicker (corderoe). The shoes took a beating in the asphalt.

We lived diagomal from the Sacred Heart Church. This meant two things. 1. Myself, Brothers Bill and Dave also would be called for serving morning mass (during the week-older kids had Sunday). 2. We would walk to early mass on a wooden street. End cuts of hard wood (soaked in tar?) paved like stone cobbles. Enyway, the Mass was in Latin and the church was beautiful. We (alterboys) got to learn some Latin. The Second War was going on in those days 1941-1945. I graduated from Sacred Heart in 1949 and from high school in 1953. The Korean War was over in 1953 but I joined the Marines and served 3 yeards. It was a teriffic experience. After that was college 1958-62, grad school 63-64- B.U.-MFA then to teach at Bishop Stang and 30 years in various schools.

April 26 - Monday - 7:58 PM

Splendid weather again- a great spring. Gentle breazes in & out clouds. Not much rain. In the ncws today- the high school shoot up. Terrible. A proof of the existantce of Evil.

Visited the people on the Cape- the Bradshaws. Everything is brand new. Splendid location. Very nice set up.

I am concerned about the decline of the quality of profecession sports among other things. Physically and mentally I feel great but with creative memory (not sure of the accuracy).

The squerills will continue to come to the bird feeder no matter how I chace them out. (I use a long stack and hit the feeder).

Rose brightens my day. of course. Besides being a very conscientios teacher and cook, Rose is a good friend. My ideas for a better tomorrow include just keep going and try to make the right decisions. Keep smiling.

Now on Monday, Wednesday and Friday I put my gym stuff in a bag and walk down to the Boys' Club. Its a mile and 1/2 down and back. I include the walk (3 miles) with the workout. At the club I do a series of exercises-I more than get my monies worth. I emphasize repite of various exercises: sit ups, push-ups, light weights (10 Ibs) in various useages. I do not push myself in this endeavor. This is followed by the sona for a short visit. Top off with a quick cold shower. There is a certain amount of banter. Some of the guys I've known for 30 & 40 years. The work out and sona are followed by a quick march home. On Tuesday, Thursday and Saturday I will take a couple of walks-again the qiuck march.

(Rose's note: the following entry was dated 4-27-99 and then crossed out and 3-4-99 written in. However, it would logically be April 27 to follow the previous entry and the short comments make chronological sense.)

April 27

A good-for-the-garden rain today. Mostly all day a steady light rain.

The business goes on in the unfortunate mess at Kosovo and serbia. It gets uglier and uglier.

May 10

Walking is very important to me. 1. It is great exercise if done right (quick march). Fortunately there are many hills in Fall River. Today walk #1 started at home, walked over to Highland Ave up Valentern St. to Elsbree St, to President St up to Robeson St. up to Hood St and left onto Greenlawn. 2. The third is the famous Somerset trip. Down Weetamoe (Princess) St. (steep!) to Main St. past the cemetary to the Brightman St Bridge. It is quite a production. Today I noticed 35 trees planted and braced along side the location where the new Road will be.

Anyway, we continue over to the 200 yr. house- and to the river. Back along the river to the bridge and cross the river again & up Brightman St. and up the hill. Weetamoe is formital and today I came up thru North Park. The tress alround are in very good condition. After supper Rose & I took a walk down President hill and down to the river with the historical surroundings. Each walk has a difference, each has a different story to tell.

May 11

Another splendid day. The sun might have been too strong. Red Sox player (Garciapara) hits two basefull home runs and one with 2 on = 10 RBI.

Tomorrow we pick up Heather at school. We borrow a vehicle from the Weissmans. (Journal suggests completing the phrase "I am excited about..." Jack writes the following in response) I would not use that word. I would say that mostly things are fine. I feel fine about things. I am concerned about Mr. Altzeit (sp.) I look it as something that happens. So far I have handled it ok. Rose has been great. Physically I feel great. Mentally- I have meory problems. I do what I can. I learn every day that in order to get something, you have to do it. (nothing for nothing)

Almost everyone and everything brightens my day. Example- I'll look at the ants at their business! My day is full of interesting occasions. "Have a good day! Good to see you! How are things going?" A good word and a smile.

Ideas for a better tomorrow: smile, read history, a good walk. Today I took three walks.

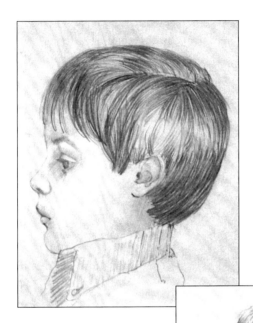

Portraits of Kevin and Heather
One of Jack's specialties was children's portraits. Kevin and Heather "sat" for their father in the early 1980s.

These next three pages are examples of Jack's word lists that he made while reading. He was fascinated by word origins and meanings.

6/10/99 WILL DURANT XXIX P647 ^{CH.}
THE Unification of Russia
I. The People P.647-650
II. The Princes of Moscow 650-653
III. IVAN THE TERRIBLE 1533-84   [278 to 9]

6/11/99

1520-66 Suleimon the Magnificent Ch. XXXI

I. AFRICAN ISLAM 1200-1566

GONFALONIER 1477 LEO   WIGHT
BETE NOIRE   CORNICE   OBSEQUY MINIVER
            OGIVE TRANSEPT PORTICO ARCH
RECUMBENT   GAUDY   RECONDITE
PEREGRINATIONS CORNICE PILASTER UBIQUITOUS
CREDENZA   PIANO   DISSIDENT
VENERY HEBDOMADAL CORNICE SHIELD
BLITHE PULLULATING ELLIPTICAL LAXITY
                PERTINACIOUS
MACARONIC   SANGUINE VENAL
    ENTOMOLOGICAL   VAUNT
                        CATACLINE
                        OBSEQUIOUS
                        ANADYOMENE
                        ESCHATOLOGY
                        CUPOLA
                        AGNOSTIC
CORNICE   EVANESCENT
ASSIDUOUS EPISTOLARY   CUPIDITY
PUISSANCE CORNICE AROMA RENUNCIATION
             ESCHATOLOGY FOSS
                        DISCURSIVE

BOCCACCIO

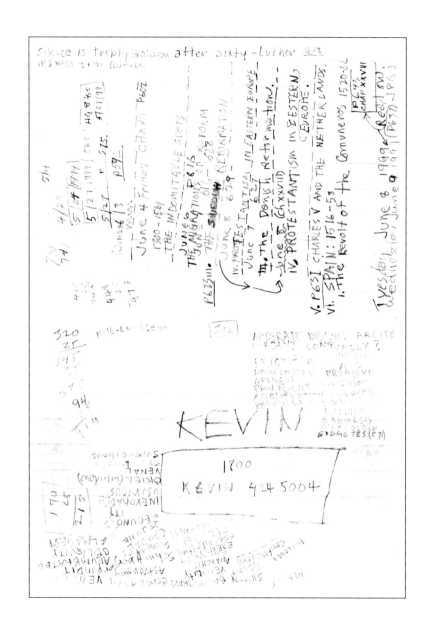

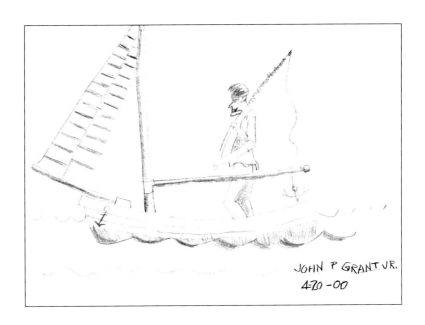

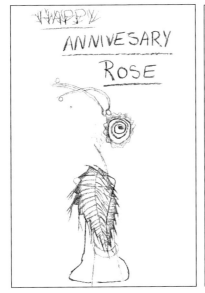

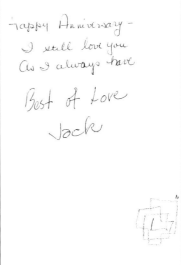

These two artworks were created after Jack entered the nursing home. The sailboat picture was actually drawn on March 20, 2000, the day he was admitted. He was either confused about the day or added it later. The anniversary card was done for June 16, 2000.

29

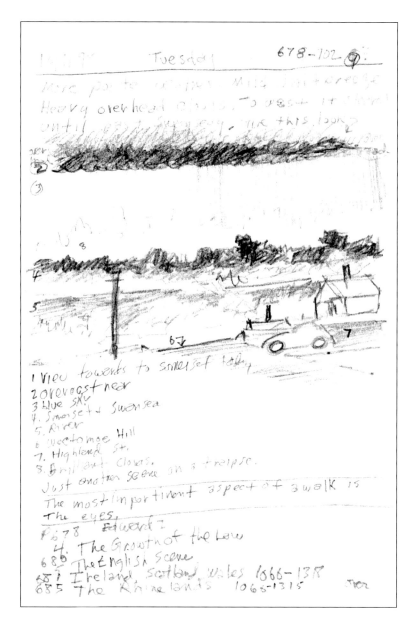

This page is from Jack's Journal, dated December 1, 1998. It is a view of Somerset, as seen from the top of North Park in Fall River.

CHAPTER FOUR

Life Goes On

After Jack left teaching on a disability retirement, things got better for him. He was less anxious, had less physical problems and was philosophical about the future. "This is what God has planned for me and there is nothing I can do about it." While I continued to work, he was glad to stay at home with his walks, his books and the garden. He helped out a lot with chores around the house and did not seem to mind. When it was frosty or snowy, he would clean the car off for me before I left for work; he said it was the least he could do! We used to joke that he was more than happy to spend me off to school. When I got home, he was happy to see me and we would set off for a walk and catch up on each other's day. He seemed content to share my teaching day vicariously.

(Caregivers Help Notes: Chore List)

In the meantime, I was trying to get myself educated on Alzheimer's. I attended a support group, caregivers' conferences, and workshops. I read everything I could get my hands on about the disease and became familiar with the Alzheimer's Association. As a teacher, I knew I needed to be pro-active and do my homework. I have always loved learning and the biggest test of my life was around the corner.

For the first few years things went well for us. We were seeing a therapist regularly, had adjusted to a lower income, saw our daughter off to college and just tried to have normal days.

Then in the late summer of 1999, Jack started complaining of bowel issues. Sometimes on a walk he would develop abdominal pain and we had to hurry home to the bathroom. He felt the urge to defecate all the time, but could not produce a movement. He said he sometimes had blood in the toilet, but I could not get him to remember not to flush to let me check. So a call was made to our primary care physician, a colonoscopy was scheduled and life threw us yet another curve ball.

CHAPTER FIVE

At Home (Stage I)

I began keeping a journal for different reasons than Jack. My journal was a place for me to record my frustrations, my complaints, my sorrows. I could not share these feelings with my best friend anymore. Sometimes I got so angry with Jack and I had to remind myself that it was Mr. Alzheimer I was mad at and not Mr. Grant. It was the disease rearing its ugly head and the journal got the brunt of my venting.

November 3, 1999

Jack had surgery for colon cancer today. The tumor was discovered during a colonoscopy in October, which was scheduled after we found blood in his stool. He had been complaining to me on and off about feeling an urge to defecate but not being able to produce anything. He has always been a prudish man and didn't like to discuss body functions, so I wasn't really aware of anything going on. Frankly, I hadn't really paid attention to his comments about how many times he went to the bathroom because I thought that if he couldn't keep track of what day it was, how could he remember how many BMs he had and when? I was quite shocked to see not only blood in the toilet but a thin, ribbon-like stool.

The tumor was fairly close to the rectum and the surgeon painted a very bleak, but realistic, picture of what was probably going to happen. He was quite sure he was going to have to do a permanent colostomy. The thought of dealing with a bag collecting feces on an Alzheimer's patient was almost more than I could endure. I knew that Jack would never be able to handle it. So when his surgeon called me from the operating room to say he was able to sew Jack's bowels back together the relief was incredible! Finally, a break for us!

November 4, 1999

When I went to see Jack at the hospital today the anesthesia was wearing off and he was ornery. He had an IV, oxygen, two surgical drains, a urinary catheter and a nasogastric tube all connected to him. He could not understand any of it and wanted OUT. We (the nurses and I) explained over and over again what had happened to him and what everything was about, but this is pretty useless to someone with AD who is also groggy from drugs. He kept tugging on the tubes, insisting that he had to get up, had to go to the bathroom, had to get dressed. Fortunately for me, the doctor had ordered aides to sit with him when I wasn't there, so it allowed me to go home to eat and sleep. Otherwise, I would have been terrified to leave him alone.

As the drugs wore off, Jack became more and more belligerent and more and more insistent on getting up. A couple of times I tried to distract him, but he began pushing me and getting angrier. Finally, while his surgeon's nurse was visiting, he got up out of bed. We both tried to get him back but he began screaming and pushing us. Nurses came running down the hall to help. He began swearing and pushing and yanked both his IV and NG tube out. There was blood everywhere. People came running from all over the unit and it took six of them to restrain him and get him back into bed.

Meanwhile, I was in the corridor crying hysterically. This was not my sweet, gentle husband in there. I was worried that the surgery was going to take away more than the cancer and it looked like I was right. The remaining vestiges of the old Jack Grant were gone too.

The only way they could keep him in bed and safe was to restrain him. With my permission, they first tried a posey jacket, but that still left his hands free to pull at tubes (they opted to leave the NG tube out but had to re-insert the IV), so later they also restrained his hands, which got him really angry. He tugged and tugged at those and finally got them off. What eventually worked were these mitten-like restraints that prevented him from using his fingers. Realize that this was all one day post-op.

I must say the hospital staff was incredible. They were professional, compassionate and kind to both Jack and me. They called in people from the psychiatric unit who were more experienced with Alzheimer's patients and they evaluated his meds to see if they could be compounding the confusion (they were). They brought in a nurse who specialized in Reiki relaxation techniques, who spent a long time with him and was wonderful in getting him calmed down.
It was a horrendous and exhausting day. I know we had to solve the bowel issue, but I am sad at how this surgery has escalated the progression of his confusion. He left more than a tumor in the operating room yesterday.

(Caregiver Help Notes: Hospitalization of an Alzheimer's Patient).

November 17, 1999

Five days post-op, Jack was eating and walking around the unit, so our doctor discharged him. Once the anesthesia wore off and we got the medication right, he was much more agreeable and easier to handle. Being back at home and in a routine helped. He kept coming to me to show me his incision and staples, saying "I've got this thing on my belly and I don't know what it is." Since he could not retain that he was recovering from surgery, I decided to stay home from work until the staples came out. I went back to work this past Monday, and today, when I got home, he told me that he had called the police. He said he was sick and should not be left alone. Trembling, I waited at the front door for the patrol car to come, trying to think about what I was going to say to the officer when he got here. Fifteen minutes went by, then twenty and still no police. I decided to punch the "last number dialed" button on our phone and heard the voice mail kick in. He had never called the police. I was relieved but shaking. I called my brother-in-law Brian and we agreed that Jack should not be left alone. Since I had already missed two weeks of school, he volunteered to stay with Jack.

I had anticipated the day when I would not be able to leave him alone anymore, but this caught me by surprise. At the end of last summer, I had sent letters to all of his friends to let them know how he was doing and to see if they would be interested in helping with day care. The response ranged from enthusiasm to hesitation to no answer. I know I was really putting their friendship on the spot! Anyway, I got their phone numbers and set up a schedule for the following week-everyone doing a four hour shift. This translates into ten time slots that have to be covered in the work week. We will see how it goes.

(Caregiver Help Notes: Letter to Volunteers & Day Care Schedule)

November 23, 1999

We drove to Mount Holyoke College today to bring Heather home for Thanksgiving. It took us two hours and fifteen minutes to get there and there was not one request for a bathroom when he is in there every fifteen minutes when we are at home. I did stop along the Mass Pike for a pit stop and he got locked in the Men's Room and could not get out. Evidently, he could not remember how to unlock the door and had to be rescued. I was really upset about it, but he was laughing off his embarrassment.

(Caregiver Help Notes-Bathrooms)

November 25-26, 1999

We get no sleep! I gave Jack 50 mg of trazodone tonight at 10 PM to go to bed and he was up and in the bathroom at 10:22 PM. I decided to record his bathroom trips:

11 PM-got up, no bathroom, 11:30 PM-flushed toilet, came out and then went right back in to toilet, 11:50 PM, 12:29 AM, 1:30 AM, 3:05 AM, 4:37 AM, 5:30 AM, 6:10 AM, 7:04 AM.

Next night: 10:32 PM bed with 50 mg trazodone, 11:37 PM, 12:07 AM, 12:35 AM with another 25 mg trazodone, 1:15 AM, 1:46 AM, 2:17 AM, 3:00 AM, gave up recording the time

November 27, 1999

Bedtime at 10:25 PM. He seems to be going to the bathroom less often. Plan to give him one 50 mg trazodone now and another if he doesn't sleep (please, God!).

December 17, 1999

Jack is very frustrated at losing his words. He loves to read and does so with a thick dictionary by his side, making lists of news words to look up later. Today he told me, "The words see me coming and they fly away." How sad and how accurate.

Other gems from this formerly articulate man:

> his description of our new niece, Sara Orton: "a pre-view of heaven"

> on seeing a flock of Canadian geese flying over head: "God is walking across my path"

> "I'm going to brush my teeth if I can find them." (He DOES NOT have dentures!!)

December 27, 1999

Jack fell asleep in a chair tonight and when he woke up he did not know me. That was the first time he did not know his own wife. I thought I would be more upset about it than I am. I knew it would happen some day.

Today Jack had his first radiation treatment for colon cancer. He had a tumor removed and his bowel resected a little over a month ago. They feel that all of the cancer was removed so the radiation is just to kill any stray cells and to keep it from coming back.

I also saw a lawyer today who specializes in elder issues and Medicaid applications. I need to be prepared if the time comes to place Jack in a facility. From the sound of it, I will lose all of his income, which will make things pretty difficult for me financially, especially with Heather having one more year of college. We cross that bridge when we get there, I guess. I had the lawyer draw up a new will for me and changed my health care proxy and power of attorney, naming the kids instead of Jack. All in all, it was a very eventful (stressful) day. Going to bed, as we need to catch sleep when it is available.

(Caregiver Help Notes: Legal Issues)

CHAPTER SIX

Stage II

———

Life was becoming more and more of a challenge. Jack was getting harder to handle, we were getting very little sleep and the disease was marching on. I was still going to work each day (I shudder to think about the quality of my teaching then with so little sleep and so much on my plate). I would come home to relieve my day care helper and begin my own sixteen hour shift. After Christmas, I had a meltdown and called the social worker from my support group. We met and placed Jack on the waiting list for a bed at Country Gardens. It was such an awful step but I knew I had to do it.

That January I started the process of applying for Medicaid with my attorney, who specialized in elder issues. The paperwork for this process is overwhelming. In 1999, the "look back" period was three years; I believe it is now five. This means finding bank records, tax returns, utility bills, and volumes of other documents while simultaneously doing my income tax returns and the financial aid forms for our daughter. Oh, yes-and teaching full time, followed by care-giving. I was beginning to lose my mind.

February 1, 2000

I have wanted to be more faithful to keeping this journal, but my day is so full it is hard to find the time. I have decided to write each night while I watch the news. Here's a typical day for me:

5:30-7:00 AM: Wake up and shower. Breakfast, make lunch. Dress and get ready for school. Small chores, laundry, run dishwasher.

7:00 AM-3:00 PM: School

3:00-4:30 PM: St. Anne's Oncology for radiation treatments (28 days in all)

4:30-10:30 PM: Supper, chores, bath and skin care for Jack, laundry, school work, general picking up around the house, possibly TV, bed!

Sleep is precious. We don't get much. Jack gets up several times a night to go to the bathroom. Sometimes he is quite confused, having trouble finding his way out of the room, to the bathroom, and back. Many nights he doesn't make it back to our room on one of his trips, ending up in Heather's bedroom instead. This was interesting when she was home for Christmas break!

I have been having an assortment of people coming in each day to stay with Jack, including his brother Brian, our son Kevin (on his day off), my sister Charlene (with new baby daughter Sara), and three of his friends, Don, Jim and Bill. My sister Carol was part of the crew while she was out of work, but unfortunately for us, she got a new job. It is too bad that she can't come anymore, because she is a nurse and definitely the one he liked best. That's funny because before AD she was not one of his favorite people!

We have five days of radiation left. Every day when I get home from work, it is a rush to get him changed and to St. Anne's.

Since he could not get himself undressed and into a johnny for the procedure without assistance, the hospital suggested that he wear sweat pants that could just be pulled down for the treatment. That makes things easier for the hospital, but EVERY DAY I have to explain why he has to change his clothes and where we are going and why we are going there. It really wears on my patience! I will be so glad when it is over. It has dominated our lives for six weeks. Jack's skin is burned and dry on his butt and he complains constantly about pain, urgency to use the toilet and so on. I am sure he is uncomfortable, but not being able to retain why it is happening and the purpose of it, only makes it worse. I'll be glad when it all heals- for both of us!

Since I last wrote, I have visited two nursing homes and have an appointment to see a third on Monday. This is heartbreaking for me, but the day of placement is getting closer and closer. Last week Jack verbally attacked me, calling me a liar and a thief. He told me to "get on a plane and fly 1000 miles from here" because otherwise he was calling the police to come and get me. I know he doesn't know what he is saying but it was still pretty scary. He is a very gentle person and it was frightening to see this "mean" side of him.

Our therapist told me I would know when it was time for placement: when my sleep is constantly disturbed, when my job is affected and when I am frequently getting sick. I have been ill three times since Christmas, which is very unusual for me. Is it time?

February 2, 2000

Things that drive me crazy:

-lost sleep, lost glasses, lost books, lost words, lost memories

-paranoia
-being accused of being a liar, thief, communist, "the other woman", when I am really exhausted from trying to be the best caregiver I can be
-sundowning that begins at 3 PM
-manic lectures about communism, politics, injustice, and slavery
-radiation treatments, diarrhea, soiled underwear, burned skin, incontinence
-being told to stay strong, stay healthy, be patient, find time for myself
-being told that I am not entitled to respite aid because I work full-time and am "only" a caregiver part-time (16 hours of the day!)
-rummaging that extends to my clothes, my books, my school papers
-"visitors" while in the bathroom
-telephone/television jealousy

February 6, 2000

What an adventure yesterday! I had gotten two pairs of knit pants for Christmas and they were a bit too long. I had been unable to find the time to take them to be shortened and finally got to go yesterday. Naturally, Jack came along for the ride. The tailor is this sweet lady who runs a drycleaners in the south end of the city. I went into the shop, got Jack seated, and said I would be right out from the dressing room. At the time his comment, "That remains to be seen." seemed odd, but I went in and got changed. The lady quickly realized that the pants hadn't been washed, so she wouldn't shorten them for me. I changed back into my other pants and got ready to leave. (As an aside, this incident was one of those little things that almost put me over the edge. I was fighting back tears in the place because I was disappointed that I would have to find another time to get there and I knew that wouldn't be easy). Just as we began to leave, Jack started to get confused and agitated about why we were there. A few other customers came in so I hurried him out to the parking lot. His confusion and agitation escalated and he refused to get into the car. He said he wanted no part of the "organization" and what was happening there. He said he was walking home! It was about 40 degrees and sunny, but he only had his spring jacket on and it is about five miles from our house. I told him it was too far, but he took off. I didn't know what to do but I got in the car and caught up to him. I pulled over and beeped the horn and he crossed the street and got in the car. I thought, "Ah, ha! Got him!" I quickly hit the power button to lock him in and took off. He soon started yelling, "Where are you taking me? Let me out of here!" I assured him that we were just going home but he called me a liar. About half a mile down the next street I had to stop at a light and he tried to get out of the car but found himself locked in (HA! I thought). But, as I started to drive again, he quickly pulled up the door lock and was out of the car and OFF! I couldn't believe it! I went to the next light, did a U-turn and he had disappeared. I drove back up Brayton Avenue, right onto Stafford Road, down to Warren and checked each street that crossed up and down but could not find him. I was frantic and at the same time amazed at how fast he had disappeared. I didn't know what to do, so I drove home and called Jack's brother Brian. He looked for him but couldn't find him either. We had decided that Brian would go to the police with a photograph of Jack and he left our house to do that, only to quickly return. He had seen Jack coming home on Robeson Street. He arrived home and had no recollection of what had happened. He just thought he had had a great walk! When I told him why I was so upset and why I was crying, he began to cry himself and said he didn't understand why he did such things.

Later that night he called me a liar again because his Irish sweater had been moved from where he thought he had left it.

This is so not like the old Jack. He would never talk to me that way in the old days.

(Caregiver Help Notes: Identification Bracelets)

February 10, 2000

On Monday I went to a nursing facility in New Bedford to meet with the social worker to consider putting Jack in adult day care. The center looked promising and after meeting with her for over an hour, we decided to try Jack on Tuesdays and Thursdays. The "fib" was to tell him he was working there as an aide. He needed a Mantoux TB test to go there, so my school nurse said she would do it for me. Yesterday we had a day of workshops scheduled at school, so the plan was to have him go to work with me, get his shot, have some breakfast and get picked up by Don at 8:45 AM. All went well until Don arrived to take him and he didn't want to go with him. We managed to get him to go but he later refused to get in Don's car after they had stopped for coffee and a muffin. I talked to Don last night and he felt that all was okay. I can't afford to alienate any of my helpers!

I have been agonizing over placing Jack in a nursing home. Sometimes he is so lucid and happy. My old husband is there. These are the times when I just can't bear to think of putting him in a home. Then he gets paranoid and calls me hateful names and can't remember who Kevin is or that this is his home and then….

I keep procrastinating about this momentous decision. My friend Donna (our school nurse whose mother has AD) said yesterday that "Husbands put their wives in nursing homes too early and wives do it too late." She has been tremendously helpful and supportive to me.

Anyway, God works in mysterious ways. Today I got home from school and there was a message from the social worker from Country Gardens Nursing Home. I called her back and she said she has a possible opening. She is going to screen Jack and one other person for this placement. This may force me to do something. This is the place where I want him to go if he must. She is going to visit us next Tuesday.

Also, I called our psychiatrist today and he called me back tonight. He told me that if Jack has another episode like getting out of the car while it is moving or another aggressive episode with me or anyone else, we can get him hospitalized under some code. This might make it easier to get him placed. He is going to document the three episodes I told him about tonight. I didn't even know this was a possibility. I hope it doesn't come to that but it does give me an out. We want to keep him from hurting himself or anyone else.

So two phone calls today that may help me to make the next painful step that I will have to take soon.

February 11, 2000

Don called me today at school at 10:15 AM and told me that Jack had just told him to get out of the house. Jack said he was going for a walk and when he got back Don had better be gone. Don didn't know what to do but I told him to go because I was afraid Jack would get too agitated if he stayed. I got coverage for my classes and came home. Jack was happy as a clam to see me, as if nothing had happened! Now I am down one less day care person. The crunch is on!

February 16, 2000

E-mail message from my sister Charlene, who helps with day care, accompanied by her infant daughter Sara.

"Jack was very sweet today. He showed me the Valentine card he got from you and told me, "She is one dynamic lady." He said he is going to keep this card because there is a lot of love in it and his name is on it and so is Rose's, so he is part of a good thing. He pointed to the note you wrote in it and said to me, "I am a little too old for that. Wait! No, I am not! It still feels great!" I told him it is good to know that and he said, "Yes, it is."

He enjoyed Sara. She smiled for him and talked a lot today.

He told me he couldn't read books with a lot of words any more. They get fuzzy on him. He said, "Hey, how are you, Jack? I am a little fuzzy" and he laughed.

He read the mail and saw John P. Grant and said, "That guy is dead. (He is referring to his father) It is supposed to be junior but that's okay. He was one tough guy. They called him 'Tough John'. He didn't back down from anyone and he had the nose to prove it." I enjoy his wittiness.

It has been a privilege to visit with him and I have enjoyed it.

Love, Charl"

February 20, 2000

Last Tuesday the nursing home social worker came for a visit. She, Jack and I sat at the kitchen table sharing a snack and a coffee. In the hour-long visit she spoke almost exclusively with Jack, who was very friendly and talkative. She was here to evaluate him for placement at Country Gardens Nursing Home (CGNH) and when she left she said he was absolutely ready. In some ways, I was tremendously relieved to have the decision made. From what was said I assumed that he would be placed in about a week to ten days. Then on Thursday I spoke to her from school and discovered that the bed she had for Jack was given to an emergency placement! I really broke down in the faculty room when I got off the phone. Joanne, a fellow teacher and friend, was there to comfort me. Later other people who have had experience with nursing homes told me this was standard procedure. It is tremendously frustrating to have finally made this decision only to have it postponed. Hopefully it won't be for long. She tells me there will be another opening this week.

On Friday Donna, our school nurse, asked me to stop by her office during third period. When I arrived, there were a few kids there, so she took me across the hall for what I thought was a private conversation in another office. When we got there three boys were in there, so I thought we would have to go somewhere else for our talk. As it turned out, these boys-Ryan, Oliver and Corey -were waiting for me. They had a big card and a bunch of flowers. I soon discovered that these three boys had been very concerned about my situation with Jack and wanted to do something to help out. What they did was go around to all of the homerooms (with administrations' permission) and take up a collection for me. I received two grocery gift certificates, an anonymous check from a parent to pay one month's mortgage and a check from the whole school for $3700! I almost died. What an incredible thing to do! To know these boys and to know they did this makes it all the more incredible. This will really help me when I lose Jack's income. It shows the kind of place this school is and has always been. Finally, something nice has happened to us.

There are many times a day when my old Jack is there and I think, "What am I doing thinking about a nursing home?" Then he will say something like "I still don't understand what this organization is all about (referring to our house) and who all these people are who work here." And I realize he might as well be at CGNH because he doesn't recognize this place as home. Tonight at supper he said, "I wish I could eat here all the time because the food is so good, but I guess I can't afford to come here all the time."

Today it was cold, bright and sunny with melting snow. We went for a walk (2 miles) and had a good time. About a half-hour after we got home he asked me to go for a walk and got really mad when I said, "No, we just went for a walk." He started yelling at me and lecturing me about selfishness.

Latest Obsessions:

> Towels, Bill Rodgers' book on running, eye glasses, wallet, Irish sweater, other sweaters, pajama bottoms, green jacket

Layers of clothes:

> Underwear, pajamas, 2 pairs of sox, corduroy pants, sneakers, flannel shirt (same one day after day), two sweaters (all worn at the same time!)

February 22, 2000

I am on vacation this week. Today we did lots of errands in the morning and then met Jack's mother, his brother Brian and sister-in-law Shirley at a local Italian restaurant for lunch. When I told him we were going to do that, his response was, "Why would I want to eat with people I don't know?" Anyway, he had a really bad time ordering his lunch, so I had to order for him. Unfortunately, everyone's entrees came out from the kitchen except his and he got really upset that everyone had a plate but him. Wouldn't you know that it would be his food that would be late? During the meal he had a lot of muscle cramping in his right hand and shared it with everyone at the table. (I thought this was very amusing since my mother-in-law is in major denial that anything is wrong with him). As we were leaving the restaurant, he escorted his mother to his brother's car and gave her a big bear hug! The rest of us were hysterical because she is not a very demonstrative person and the "new" Jack was forcing her to be affectionate.

Late this afternoon I was doing some sewing in our bedroom and he came in and started doing some major rummaging in our room. He was ranting and raving about all of the things that are missing and the stealing that was going on. Many of the items he came across were his own possessions, but he did not recognize them and talked about how thieves left their things in place of his.

Last night he slept with four sweaters under his pillow. Currently, there are all kinds of clothes under his pillow and mine. He started going through Heather's things yesterday. I had moved some of my clothes into her room hoping they would be safe but nothing is off limits in here anymore. The other day I found one of my credit cards in his wallet. He has hidden Kevin's mail in his (Jack's) bureau under his clothes. What surprises are in store for us when he leaves and we get to clean out his things?

(Caregiver Help Notes: Eating Out)

February 27, 2000

Jack went out for a walk over an hour ago. I am trying not to panic but he seems to be gone a long time, especially since he had to sit down during mass this morning because he was tired. At noon he told me he was going for a walk and set out twice only to come back almost immediately each time. It was almost as though he got out there and forgot he was taking a walk. Finally, he left to go the third time around 12:30 PM.

Well, he just arrived and told me he had walked to Swansea! He ran in and went up to the bathroom. I just heard a small shout from the room but nothing more. Lately he is full of grunts and groans.

It is beautiful outside. They expect we might set a temperature record today. It would have been a good day to get lost, I guess. At least he wouldn't be freezing.

His behavior gets more and more bizarre. The other day he seemed bored, so I asked him to vacuum our bedroom. He did but then spent the next TWO (yes!) hours yelling at me about how insulting the chores are that I give him. People give him jobs and then say, "See you later, slave! I'm going out to have a good time." He got into a huge discussion about slavery and people taking advantage of others. The entire time I tried to just sit there and let him rage. Once in a while he would leave the room and I would think, "Finally, it's over." But then he would come back in and start up again. Some of it was really difficult to listen to but I tried to put on my thick skin and not be hurt by the words. Easier said than done! It was Mr. Alzheimer talking to me and not my Jack.

He has always been one to save memorabilia-notes, cards, ticket stubs, and so on, and now he has taken them all out to read and display. I am finding notes that I put in a lunch 20 years ago tucked inside a picture frame on the wall or held by a magnet on the fridge. It is so sad- these bits of his life that he proudly displays even when he can't remember the people or the time they represent. He is hanging out his memories.

I met with my lawyer on Wednesday to sign my new will, health care proxy and power of attorney and then we looked at Medicaid. She thinks there will be no problem getting approval. She is going to try to get them to give me some of Jack's income to live on. In the meantime, it cost me $650 for that visit and I had already paid her $300. (I would come to realize this was money well spent.)

That morning I opened a safety deposit box and my own checking account at the bank. The manager there talked me into the checking account, which I did not want, but it turned out to be a good idea because later the lawyer said I should have separate accounts for Jack's expenses and mine.

The attorney told me she would contact the nursing home to tell them it was a "go" for Jack to be placed, but I also called myself, only to find that the social worker wasn't in. I left a voice mail and was a bit upset because we were going to be away all of the next day visiting Heather at school. I hoped that she would call me either that night or the next. By 8:30 PM on Thursday night there was no call, so I called a friend whose husband is a resident at the nursing home. She told me she thought that I had changed my mind about putting Jack there because someone else took the bed intended for him. She was quite upset when I told her the bed was given to someone else and even more upset to hear that I was told that someone else would be leaving to make a place for Jack. She felt this couldn't be true. There are only six men there now-her husband, the new man and four others. She couldn't imagine any of them leaving. This caused a sleepless night for me! I finally called the nursing home Friday morning and spoke with both social workers. Supposedly the opening is still coming. We scheduled a medical needs assessment for tomorrow after school with a nurse from Bristol Elder Services. I'm going to tell Jack she is coming because of his bowel problems. I have turned into a very polished liar.

(Caregiver Help Notes: Post Office and Safety Deposit Boxes)

CHAPTER SEVEN

Nursing Home Placement

March 2, 2000

The medical assessment went well. A couple of times Jack got upset with the questions such as, "Can you prepare a meal? Can you dress yourself?" I believe he was thinking that we were implying that he is stupid. Many times he insisted that he could do something independently when it doesn't happen at all. Hopefully the nurse picked up on this.

When I called the social worker on Monday to tell her that the Bristol Elder nurse was coming that day, she expressed surprise at how soon it was happening. THEN she told me that Jack also needs a physical! It is really frustrating to get these surprises thrust upon me! I quickly called our primary care doctor's office only to find that they are closed. I called again on Tuesday morning and they graciously took us at 2:30 that day. Mind you, all of this is going on while I am trying to teach all day.

It was a bittersweet visit with Dr. Sorial. I could tell by his reaction to Jack that he was shocked at the level of his deterioration. He told him that he looked very thin and that while he was otherwise healthy, his memory was very bad. Jack launched into his philosophy of life and the frailty thereof and how there was no point in getting upset about something you couldn't do anything about. Then he told Dr. Sorial that he didn't have to worry about it because he had me to take care of him; that I did a terrific job because I loved him and that he loved me very much. He soon had me crying and I'm sure Dr. Sorial was close to tears, as well. When we came out of the exam room, the office staff saw all of our faces and I thought they were going to start crying too.

The past couple of days Jack has been really with it- sleeping better, less diarrhea, less rummaging. Then today he took two long walks by himself while Brian was here doing day care, including one to the Boys' Club, which got Brian upset because he went so far and was gone so long while under his care. When I got home from school, we went for a walk and he seemed fine. Back at home after our walk, he sat down for one of his famous talks about his sweaters and getting them to a safe place. Then he went on and on about all kinds of disjointed things that I couldn't make heads or tails of. I just sat and made believe I was listening. Brian told me later on the phone that he does the same thing while he's here during the day.

After supper we sat down to watch the news and he fell asleep in the chair. About 7 PM he woke up really confused and started talking about a little boy who died. It was very weird. I had no idea who he was talking about. He said he was very tired, so I talked him into going to bed. Upstairs he was almost crying and said when he gets sick he feels like a little boy and can't find God. I gave him a Trazadone and said a prayer for a good night. He's been up there for over two hours now but has gotten up several times to use the bathroom. He does go back to bed each time.

The original bed at CGNH was given to a man named Rocco who was an emergency admission from an assisted living facility. I was told today that he was evaluated to go back to assisted living and if he does, Jack will get that bed after all. The delays are maddening.

I got a checklist in the mail today of the things the Medicaid people claim they still need for our application. Will the paperwork ever be done? Some of the items have been provided not once but twice already! Someone said this whole process is so frustrating so that you will give up on the whole thing. But what choice do I have?

(Caregiver Help Notes: Nursing Home Placement)

March 4, 2000

I go around with a lump in my throat all the time. As placement approaches, I torture myself with thinking, "This is the last time we will go out for a bagel together (or to church or grocery shopping)."

It was a beautiful, sunny, mild day today. I decided to drive down to Horseneck Beach for a walk. Jack loves the place. It was cold but absolutely beautiful. There were about eight other people there, so we basically had the whole beach to ourselves. The sky was so blue and the beach so pristine. I found a tiny sand dollar about the size of a dime (a sand dime!) and lots of beach glass, including a piece that looked to me like an angel's wing. On the way home Jack said, "I want to keep coming down here for years and years." The lump appears in my throat.

March 5, 2000

My sister Carol came by today with a lottery ticket. She stayed about fifteen minutes. After she left, Jack ranted and raved about how he won't put up with people making fun of Catholics! Where does this stuff come from? Nothing remotely related to that came up in our conversation.

We did three walks today and some yard work. Jack should sleep well tonight! He has been going to the bathroom a lot. I hope it won't be a bad night. He has spent a lot of time going through his sweaters. He talks and talks about taking them with him when he goes "home".

Today Jack said, "I know what's wrong with me. I left my memory on a bus somewhere."

March 6, 2000

My husband doesn't remember our son's name. At this writing, Kevin is twenty-four years old and works in the kitchen at a local country club. Jack can retain Kevin's job description but for some reason insists on calling him Kenny. He also insists on giving "Kenny" credit for all of the cooking around here. Tonight he said," The meals around here are really good. That Kenny has a delicate touch." It has become a standing joke between Kevin, Kenny and me. We have to find our humor when and where we can.

The other day when we walked the beach, Jack collected rocks, pieces of shells and beach glass. They have been artfully arranged on a piece of paper towel on the kitchen counter since Sunday. At supper tonight he told me he wants to take them when he goes…

No news from the nursing home today. This is NOT a case of no news is good news. I'm beginning to doubt that he will ever be placed. One part of me is happy about this, but I'm not sure my nervous system can handle this.

Jack constantly talks of future plans- to get a new pair of running shoes and begin running again, to re-join the Boys' Club, to plant trees in the backyard, to go to the beach this summer.

At supper he talked of a desire to revisit Ireland. This all makes me quite sad. What will the future really be for him?

March 7, 2000

I have been very down in the dumps today. I got into the car outside of school at 2:30 and started sobbing but had to drive away so that the students wouldn't see me. I called the social worker today and she wasn't in- so no news since last Friday. I looked at my calendar at lunchtime and realized it was three weeks ago yesterday since she told me she would take Jack and he is still at home. I am really depressed-wanting him to go and feeling bad about it- and yet I have no place to send him.

I came home and he and Bill Golden were sitting in the sun in chairs on the porch. They broke into applause as I drove into the driveway. What a welcoming committee! Then Jack and I went for a walk to get a coffee and cookie. We did almost three miles in silence; something felt funny. We got home and Jack immediately began rummaging upstairs and in the hall closet. His green jacket was on the back of a chair in the dining room and he came in to get it. He then launched into a lecture about stealing. He was going to call a lawyer to get the people who keep taking his jacket and so on. It was about half way through this twenty-minute "sermon" that I realized he was really giving a lecture to a class. He was using his version of "legalese", talking about presenting evidence to support his claim to the defense and the Commonwealth of Massachusetts. At the end he said, "Any questions? Thank you very much." He put his jacket away upstairs and I got up to make supper. Then he went looking for the jacket again and couldn't find it. I began to help him with the search and couldn't find it at first but finally found it under his pillow. I tried to distract him to go down to eat supper but he began part II of the lecture at the table, only this time we were evidently in an English courtroom. We were told to give testimony to do the right thing in honor of the Queen and for the good of her majesty's England. WOW! I wish I could record one of these sessions. As a scientist, it makes me wonder how all of these plaques and tangles in his brain can make my husband forget that he is in his own home and who his son is but at the same time he can come up with all of this verbiage that he never would have used pre-A.D. It would be fascinating if I wasn't so emotionally connected to the situation.

A little while after this happened he asked me if Rose would be stopping by today and I asked him who I was. He looked at me and started laughing, "Oh! There you are!"

March 10, 2000

I got a call yesterday, during my Bioethics class, from the social worker at CGNH. Jack's bed will be ready on Monday. I had to leave my class and go out into the corridor to compose myself to return to a lecture about abortion, no less! Get me off this emotional roller coaster!

I later spoke with her and got details of when to go and what I need to do. When I got home from school, Charlene and baby Sara were here and Jack had had a good day. We went for a three-mile walk, stopping for coffee and a cookie at "our" bakery. We had a pretty good evening. I started playing head games with myself: this is one of the last times we will do this… he's not ready to go…look how normal he is today.

Today is a bonus day off from school and yet Jack had me up by 6:20 AM. In the forty minutes I've been up, I started collecting evidence that he is NOT normal:

-insisting on keeping his pajamas on under his clothes
-feces and soiled underwear all over the bathroom

-announcing that his Irish sweater was stolen during
the night
-finding dirty dishes in the cupboards while making
breakfast

So now I will play that head game today, trying to convince myself that placement in a nursing home is the right decision.

Last night in bed before we fell asleep he told me he wants to get his sweaters out of this building and take them home. He said, "I can take one out at a time under my jacket and no one will know."

March 12, 2000

A list of lasts:

-last mass together at our parish church
-last walk together in the neighborhood
-last Saturday morning bagel breakfast, followed by
last grocery shopping
-last coffee and cookie at the bakery
-last night sleeping side by side
-last goodnight kiss

Today was a raw, gloomy Sunday. It seemed appropriate for Jack's last day at home. We went to 10 AM mass and he reached over and held my hand and told me that he loved me. This is so uncharacteristic of him- a public display of affection- in church, no less!

We had a pretty good day. Since it was so rainy, I suggested going out to do a little shopping and then we stopped for ice cream. He got a bit grumpy about waiting for the ice cream to come-the same complaint as when we went out for supper on Friday night. I don't know if it is because his sense of time is all mixed up or if he is just turning into a grouchy old man, but he is really impatient these days.

Many people called today to say they are thinking of us and praying for us: Brian, Charlene, and my friend Maureen. Another friend, Donna, came by with a supper. It is so good to know that I have so many friends and so much support.

I am very nervous about tomorrow. I pray that Jack will surprise me and settle in at CGNH without any problems. I don't want too much, do I?

One of the things Jack carries around all the time is a Swiss Army pocketknife. I thought this would not be a good thing to bring tomorrow, so I confiscated it today and hid it. Ironically, tonight he took a shower and hid his wallet before he got in and now we can't find it-we looked everywhere! He's going to be upset to go without that so I hope we do find it.

(I finally found Jack's wallet about three months after he moved to the nursing home. Living alone now, the stack of towels in the bathroom never got down to the bottom until our daughter came home from college. Getting out of the shower one night, I reached up to take a towel down from the shelf and got knocked in the head by something! Looking down, it was Jack's wallet that he had folded into the last towel in the pile!)

March 21, 2000

Jack went into Country Gardens Nursing Home on March 13. I stayed home from school that day and took him with me to do errands, have coffee and so on. We stopped at the nursing home on the pretense of delivering some papers to a friend. I was a nervous wreck. We entered right into the Alzheimer's unit and had to stand there waiting for a social worker. It was probably only ten minutes but it felt like forever. Finally, both she and the activity director, Donna, arrived. Donna invited Jack to go with her and I went with the social worker to do all of the paper work. I really had a hard time holding it all together. When we were finished, I handed over two shopping bags of Jack's clothes I had hidden in the car the night before and drove off sobbing. It was really heartbreaking. I did not go back in the unit because I really could not face him and they had told me this was the best way anyway. I really felt like I was abandoning him. Later that day Jack's brother, Brian, and I went to tell my mother-in-law the news. At close to eighty-nine, this was difficult for her to handle and she did as she has done all along- she went into major denial. Now, one week later, she finally called to ask how he is doing, but kept changing the subject when I tried to tell her.

Tuesday I went back to school and spent most of the day crying. Everyone wanted to know how it went, but it was so difficult to respond over and over and not cry. In between my weeping I had to pull it all together and teach my classes! It was terrible! Then I left school for my first visit with Jack. I was dreading the reception I was going to get from him and cried all the way there (I had called the night before and they told me he was walking around with his coat and hat on waiting for me to come and get him). Anyway, I walked in and he spied me and started crying and cheering and hugging me. He was just so happy to see me. There was no anger, no recriminations, NO ASKING TO GO HOME! I was flabbergasted-and relieved! I stayed for a couple of hours and then told him I had schoolwork to do and he said, "Fine. When will I see you again?" I couldn't get over how easy it was. I talked to my physician/brother-in-law Ken a couple of days later and he said his not asking to go home probably means that he was ready to be there.

Every day seems to get better and easier. I am crying less and less each day. Yesterday as I was leaving he asked me to out for a drink. When I told him we couldn't do that he said, "No, I didn't think so" and laughed. The day before he was really upset about me leaving and kept me there by proposing marriage. When I informed him that we have been married for twenty-seven years, he was so happy! This memory loss isn't so bad sometimes.

Today when I visited we went out of the unit to listen to music and to sing along with the piano player. He went along with it for about half an hour and then started talking about being in a prison; how he could not get out any of the doors or leave the place. He started to get agitated, so I suggested a walk and took him back to the unit. As we got through the doors, he looked around and said "See, this is better." Later, sitting in his room, he told me that today was the first day that he was comfortable there. So one minute it is a prison and the next minute he seems happy. I guess I have to learn not to put too much stock into anything he says. Go with the flow.

The nursing staff cannot get Jack to shower, so on Sunday they let me get him in there. I'm going to try again tomorrow (Wednesday) and if that works, I will give him a shower on those two days. They seem to have gotten him to change his clothes at least. He was wearing layers and layers of the same clothes day after day, with his pajamas underneath. They get him into a new, clean outfit now each day.

The first two nights he got up in the middle of the night and was disoriented. He then began yelling for the police and woke up a lot of the residents. They have altered his medication and he seems a lot less agitated.

(Caregiver Help Notes: Visiting the Nursing Home)

March 23, 2000

The weather was beautiful today and I rushed to the nursing home with coffee and cookies to have a picnic with Jack in the garden. We sat on a bench in the sun and had the whole place to ourselves. It was really nice. While we were out there a flock of Canadian geese flew overhead in a big V, honking away. It was quite a sight!

The activities director, Donna, told me that Jack has been very helpful to her- painting tulip stems and leaves on the windows in the dining room to complete the paper tulips the residents made to hang there.

Today they made sauce and meatballs for an Italian dinner they are all going to have tomorrow.

March 24, 2000

Our daughter Heather went to the nursing home for the first time today (home from college for spring break). I was worried about how both she and Jack would handle it. When he saw her he said, "I know who you are, I just can't remember your name." We went out into the garden for coffee and cookies to enjoy the sunshine. He had us laughing every five minutes with joking and silly comments. We spent two hours talking, reading magazines, listening to music. All and all I think it went well. When we left Jack was pretty matter of fact about it.

I worry that Heather is being too stoic about all of this. We cried together last night when she got home. She told me that I don't have to be strong all the time. Thank God somebody is finally saying that to me.

March 28, 2000

Kevin and I arrived at the nursing home yesterday to find my husband "holding court" in the activities room. He was painting a tree on a window as part of a spring scene-carrying on a conversation with himself about how to go about it. Every now and then he would crack a joke and have us all laughing. Then he demanded some black paint to add shading to the tree, which he proceeded to do. One of the ladies across the room (painting has become a spectator sport!) started yelling at him to stop. "Trees don't have black in them! Stop! You are ruining that tree!" she yelled. It was really comical. Jack was having a great time and our son Kevin and I felt so good watching him enjoy himself.

The nurses tell me that he is "delightful". He has taught them how to salute a la Marine Corps and entertains them with lectures and stories.

One problem they have with him is getting him to do personal care- changing into clean clothes, shaving, showering, etc. I try to do what I can when I am there. I planned to get him into the shower on Wednesday and Sunday, but this past Sunday he argued with me, so I let it go and got him in there yesterday instead. He needs lots of cues and encouragement to get the job done. I know he would not be able to do it himself and he certainly would not shower in front of another woman (a nurse). We have a meeting on Thursday to discuss his comprehensive care plan. Maybe this will come up and they will have some suggestions.

(Caregiver Help Notes: Caregiving After Placement)

March 30, 2000

I met with the care team today: nurses Wendy and Judy, CNA Maureen, activity director Donna, social worker Sarah and a secretary. All thought Jack was adjusting well to the nursing home. There were some minor complaints about him not joining in at times (not unusual for Jack anyway) and with his personal care. No surprises.

We later went to listen to music and to sing along and he did fine.

April 3, 2000

I reach for a mug to make tea and automatically take two down to the counter before I remember that I am alone. The loneliness is difficult at times. I did not go to the nursing home today. My doctor advised taking a day off this week to see if I could handle it. Kevin went in my place. Instead I came right home from school and went for a walk. I fought tears for three miles and now they are about to brim over. I miss him so much! I told someone I have become a widow without a funeral.

Our friends of twenty-six years, the Donahues, drove down from Wethersfield, Connecticut on Saturday. They took me out to lunch and then we went to see Jack. I had warned them that he might not recognize them, but when he saw us, he wrapped all three of us in his arms and gave us one big hug. We showed them all around the facility and had a good visit. Bob Donahue and I were crying when they left. Good friends.

On the weekend Jack talked a lot about the future-starting a running program, going to the beach, etc. I begin plotting in my head. Where can we go to the beach other than Horseneck since I would have to drive through Fall River to get there?

Maybe Newport would work. I think he would be happy with that.

April 7, 2000

I visited Jack today and in the two hours I was there he went from being very unhappy there- the place is a prison, Nazis work there, and so on-to what a great place it is-the people are so nice, the food is great, the rooms are so pretty. He told me that most of the time he is really happy but sometimes he is really sad and cries. Yesterday the nurse told me he was ranting and raving at everyone in the morning and then sat down for breakfast and started crying and apologized to everyone.

Many months ago he said to me, "I wish you could get into my brain and see what this is like from my side." I wish I could do just that to help me understand what it does feel like. It must be very frightening to not know what is what from one fifteen minute segment of time to another; to not know who all of these people are who are all around you.

The nurses and activity director have gotten Jack to do some drawing, so I brought in a sketchpad, pastels and some other art supplies. Today when I came in, I looked everywhere and couldn't find any of these things. I was so annoyed that they had lasted only one day! Then I looked around again and found the pastels hidden in his clothes. The sketch pad was between the wall and his nightstand. He sabotages himself!

I had heard that many things get stolen in nursing homes, but I now know that they all take each other's things and hide their own things and none of it is malicious. They don't remember which room is their own and which closet is theirs. If they can't remember what day it is or where they are or their kids' names, how can they tell that the shirt they are wearing doesn't belong to them?

When President Reagan announced that he had Alzheimer's disease we were just getting into the disease ourselves. I remember how Nancy's description of "a long goodbye" really struck me as so poignant and so sad. When I go to the nursing home and see the others there, confined to wheelchairs or beds, unable to walk or talk, I ask myself if that is where we are heading. I'm sure Nancy Reagan would understand exactly my preference to have Jack die of something else without a goodbye. A heart attack would have been so much kinder for both of our husbands.

April 14, 2000

Jack was so positive when I visited today. He was happy about the food, the garden, the blue sky. Some days he depresses me with talk of prison, the Nazis (the staff!) and even suicide. He was quite upbeat today, smiling and friendly and pleasant to everyone. Several days this week I was a coward when it was time to go. One day he fell asleep on his roommate's bed while he held my hand and I extricated myself and tiptoed out and went home. Yesterday he walked out while we were reading in his room and didn't come back. When I went looking for him, he was on his way to supper, so I ducked out. Today I left while he was in the bathroom! It is so much easier than the guilt trip he puts me on when I try to leave and say goodbye. But I feel so guilty anyway for being so sneaky. A friend at work reminded me that he quickly forgets if he gets mad or is disappointed about my going.

I am leaving tomorrow morning for three days in Maine to visit my sister Pat. I won't be able to see Jack for two days and that will be another guilt trip but I am so looking forward to going and getting away from Alzheimer's for a few days. I will go right to the nursing home on Monday when I get back. Lots of other people plan to visit Jack while I am gone so he won't be lonely.

Since Jack has gone into the nursing home (four weeks), he has "lost" two jackets, a hat, a book, his glasses and a sweater. This is very frustrating- especially his jackets and glasses. One jacket only lasted one day! I am convinced that he is hiding them somewhere. I just wish I could find his hiding place! They are no where in his room. I am going to try to do a search next week when I am off and have more time. If we can locate his hiding places at least we will know where to look in the future.

April 20, 2000

Today I sat in the warm sunshine on my porch taking in the sights and sounds of a beautiful spring day. The daffodils and tulips are all in bloom and I thought, "Jack would love to be here so much." Later I spent two hours doing yard work and thought how much he would want to be here helping me if he could. So many losses.

I got to the nursing home today at 2 PM and found Jack sound asleep sitting on a couch in the common area near the nurses' station. There was all kind of noise around him but it took me quite a while to wake him. He was really disoriented and wobbly on his feet. It scared me a bit at first.

I wanted to take him out for ice cream and when I asked the nurse she said she thought it would be a good idea since he had had a "depressed" morning. Anyway, he was more than happy to go and we drove to Somerset for cones of chocolate ice cream, which we ate sitting in the grass looking at the swans on the Cole's River. It was a pretty day and he had a good time. We went for a ride before returning to the nursing home and as we approached the building he said, "Oh! There's my school! It's a great place- they will let you in, but they won't let you out!"

There is a farm that we can see from Jack's room with many cows in a field on the other side of a stone wall. He constantly talks of taking a walk to see the cows, so before we went back into the building we did just that. He was thrilled to see the animals up close. Along the way, we found a dollar bill in the grass and he asked me if he could keep it because he has no money.

Think of how little it takes to make him happy these days- a cone of chocolate ice cream, some cows and a one-dollar bill!

April 21, 2000

I got to Country Gardens late today due to a dentist appointment. As soon as I got into the building several people informed me that there had been an "incident" earlier today with Jack. He was very upset and yelling about Korea. Something about our country sending seventeen-year-old boys to fight for no good reason. It evidently took quite a bit to calm him down. Donna, from activities, managed to get him to sit with her and listen to classical music.

He told me later that he wanted to call me but couldn't remember my name. He seemed fine while I was there but I am worried that he is suffering from depression. I plan to talk to the psychologist next week.

One of the other men in the unit is very scary at times. He gets right in your face and yells in words that are almost impossible to understand. His normal state is quite agitated and the staff frequently has to redirect him. Most of the ladies are afraid of him and I will often take him by the hand to remove him from what looks like a potential altercation. My daughter tells me that I am asking for it, but I know that somewhere in there was once a nice man. I know this because every day his wife comes in to visit and she is a sweetheart. A lady like this would not have married such an ornery, nasty man nor would she come every day to walk with him, holding his hand and telling him that she loves him. Mr. Alzheimer has stolen her husband just as he took mine. I wish everyone could have known the old Jack as I have.

April 29, 2000

Heather and I went to visit Jack on Easter. They had a dessert buffet from 2-4 PM, so after having a nice dinner at my sister's, we went to see him. Initially, we had a great visit but as we sat talking, he became more and more agitated, talking about a string of totally unrelated subjects. Not much of it made any sense.

We got him down to his room away from the other people and the noise to try to quiet him down. It seemed to work a bit but wasn't entirely successful. Since it was getting close to when we wanted to leave, I told him that I had to give Heather a ride somewhere and had to leave temporarily. He bought the story, so we left. Evidently he kept the thought that I would be back because the agitation continued after we left. Later that night another patient fell (a man) and Jack went to help him up. Of course, the nurses told him not to help- to let them take care of it. He said, "This is my friend- I will help him!" When the nurses insisted that they help, he shoved one of them away. This type of behavior is deemed combative, so I was called about 8:30 PM (via a voice mail message). The social worker was also called and had to go back to work to see what was going on. She told me that by the time she got there a male relative of one of the patients was sitting with him having juice and crackers and all was well.

(Caregiver Help Notes-Holiday Visits).

At the time this was going on, I was stuck in traffic on the Mass Pike, returning from bringing Heather back to Mount Holyoke College. I didn't actually hear about it until Monday evening when I listened to my voice mail. In the meantime, I had called the social worker from work on Monday and met with her before I saw Jack. We agreed that he is depressed and they started him on Risperdal. A week later things seem to be better.

Yesterday the social worker and several of the staff told me Jack was very funny that day and had everyone laughing. I took him out for coffee and pastry and we had a nice visit. As we were leaving the building, we walked by a statue in the courtyard. It is of a nude woman pouring water from an urn. Her backside faces the building while she looks toward the highway. As we approached the statue he said, "Madame that is NOT your best side!"

Today we planted pansies in the garden and in a couple of containers that we put on the porch. It is amazing how much he has lost, including his gardening skills. He had no clue about what to do in the garden.

May 5, 2000

We had a very warm day today and Jack spent part of it turning over the soil in one of the raised beds at the home.

June 16, 2000

It is our 27th anniversary today. We have always celebrated our anniversary by going to a nice restaurant but I knew that this was out of the question this year. Jack loves flowers so I bought a big bunch and made a beautiful arrangement. I had told Donna (activities) that Jack would be upset if he didn't have a card for me, so she spent two days working on one with him. He tried to draw a rose in a vase on the cover, but the result was very bizarre-almost like a Picasso! It is so sad to see how much he has lost, including his talents in art. (See Jack's artwork)

The nursing home had an anniversary party for us- a cake, with the card and flowers for me (from Jack). Many of the staff and residents came, including the social worker, nurses, even the administrator of the facility. It was really nice of them.

I had thought ahead to bring our wedding album and everyone enjoyed looking at the photos of our 1973 "hippy" wedding.

June 28, 2000

I went to the beach alone today, for the first time in twenty-seven years. Jack so loved the beach. I wish I could take him but it would be a pretty dangerous thing to do- too many people, so easy to get lost, the issue of the water. Several years ago, early into AD, Jack got very confused on the beach. He went for his usual run along the beach and, trying to time it right, I watched for his return. As he approached our spot on the beach, I went down to meet him, but he kept right on running. Then I started running after him, but could not catch up. From a distance, I watched horrified as he approached a woman sitting in a chair, sat down on her blanket and proceeded to help himself to a drink from her cooler! All of this time, she was yelling at him to go away. By the time I got there, my legs were like jelly and I was a nervous wreck. When I managed to get his attention, he realized he was in the wrong place and we both apologized to the woman. After I got him back to our chairs and occupied in a book, I went back and explained his condition to the woman. She felt badly about yelling at him and was very understanding. Many times after that I had to explain and apologize about his "bad" behavior. Everyone was really nice about it once they understood. Many people only think of Alzheimer's disease as a memory problem and are not aware of the behavioral issues.

I have volunteered with a piping plover conservation project so that when I go to the beach I have something to do. These shore birds are on the endangered species list. I have four sites to check for numbers of birds, birds on the nest versus hatched, fences to check and repair. I'm officially called a "plover warden!" We had a strong line of thunderstorms come through last night and they must have coincided with high tide because the wrack (washed up seaweed and debris) line was inside the protected areas and had pulled down many of the fences. I spent almost 2 hours fixing them. I almost didn't have time to miss Jack.

We have had two care plan meetings since Jack has gone in. Both times we discussed his problems with personal care. He does not shower, shave or change his clothes unless I get him to do it. Once in a while they get him to shave but otherwise it is a struggle. His feet are a mess because I don't think he changes his socks and keeps them on day and night. One of the aides showed me how to do his foot care which I have been doing because he is so much more cooperative with me.

My doctor wants me to stop doing any of his care because it is not my job anymore. I read that caregivers have a hard time giving up their role once they have done it for so long. When I think of it, there are three wives and three husbands who come in everyday to feed and help care for their spouses. One man is there almost all day.

The activities director got Jack to help with the vegetable garden. They put in tomatoes and eggplants and today we added green beans. My "master gardener" could not tell a good plant from a weed, could not remember how to stake a tomato plant nor recognize that a droopy plant needed water.

July 26, 2000

I am writing while sitting on the porch of the Appalachian Mountain Club headquarters at Pinkham Notch in the White Mountains of New Hampshire. This was one of our favorite vacation destinations- summer for camping and hiking and winter for snow-shoeing and cross country skiing. We tried to come up here at least twice a year, more often if we could. Jack and I hiked the Range Hike- a one week backpack along the summits, staying in AMC huts, the summer after we were married. When the kids came along, we continued to hike, carrying them in a backpack or snuggli. When they were big enough to hike, they got their own little packs to carry a drink, a snack and a teddy bear. As teenagers, they carried thirty-pound packs and left the old folks in the dust.

I am camping at Moose Camp in North Conway. We have been camping here for about 25 years. It is a very quiet, very primitive camp along the Saco River. It was really difficult to come here alone-there are so many memories of the place that I shared with Jack. We camped here last year and I knew it would be our last time here together. We almost had to come home after two days because he got so confused about where we were and why we were there, but I talked to him and he stuck it out. We had a great week together and he really enjoyed it. But, looking back, I wonder what I really put him through getting him to stay there. It must have been confusing and even terrifying at times for him to wake up in the middle of the night in a tent. This was only three months prior to his bowel surgery (we had not yet had the colonoscopy or diagnosis of colon cancer at this time). We had to make frequent trips to the latrine, day and night. I now appreciate so much what an effort he must have made for me to see that week through.

Many of my friends were upset that I was going camping alone. One even offered me a gun for protection! But I knew that I would be going to a safe place and would have familiar people around me in camp. The only real danger to me has been the emotional ghosts that sneak up on me at unexpected times and make me cry for my hiking partner who will never hike with me again. But life goes on for me and it would be wrong to give up on it and all the things I enjoy. I have to face the new challenges that the loneliness brings to me.

July 27, 2000

Heather and one of her friends have joined me camping. Tonight we had dinner at Pinkham Notch. They serve dinner family style-all you can eat- hiker's grub! You sit at a table with 10 or 11 other hikers and meet all of these interesting people. That night, across from the girls, sat a couple from Israel. Max and Ruth emigrated there from the US. He was in New Hampshire working as a naturalist (astronomy) for the summer. They appeared to be a well-kept 70 something. Heather and her friend had a fascinating evening with them. I sat at the other end of the table with another single woman, who was hiking with a bunch of Boy Scouts, and a couple (male and female friends). This woman was telling me that it was her first hiking experience- her friend had convinced her to try it. She confided that she had lost her husband last year at age 49. She had decided to go out and try all new things- a new life. I told her about Jack and she said she didn't know how I could do all the things we did together without him. I don't want a new life- I want my old one with him. Who knows which one of us has it right? We all have to do what is best for us.

August 8, 2000

I went for a walk tonight on a sultry summer evening. Before I got off my block I met the assistant from my dentist's office who stopped to ask about Jack. We parted with her promising to keep us in her prayers. Two minutes later I met a woman walking her dog. Our sons went all through school together and her ex-husband had had Jack for a teacher. She, too, asked about Jack, so I went through the whole nursing home/cancer story as I hadn't seen her in a long time and needed to bring her up to date. At one point I looked over at her and she was wiping tears from her cheeks. I tried not to make eye contact with her for the rest of our conversation so that I wouldn't cry, too. Well, on it went for my entire walk. I met another woman-another concerned inquiry-and then the wife of a friend of Jack's, who invited me to join them on their deck for iced tea, which I did. Back on my route to get home before dark, I met three women walking, one of whom I knew by sight from church. "How's your husband doing?" one more time! All the ladies knew someone with AD, so I was on the receiving end of much compassion and understanding. So a forty minute walk took me an hour and a half tonight, but I came home with a heart full of positive feelings for and from all of those good people out there who really do care.

Today when I visited Jack he told me that he had to get busy writing some things for his father to give to him tonight. Yesterday he told me he was going to look through some books to find something to read to his father. My father-in-law has been gone for almost 24 years. Many of the other patients talk about getting home to their parents-"My mother and father are waiting for me." But this is a first for Jack. I guess a few more years of regression have taken place.

Jack has forgotten how to go to Mass. We went yesterday at the home and he didn't know his prayers anymore. This is from a guy who once knew the whole mass in Latin and sang for the bishop as a young boy. Every time we responded to the priest, he thought I was talking to him and asked what I said. He kept saying that he didn't understand me or what was going on. I feel badly about this because he loved going to church.

August 9, 2000

Today is Jack's 65th birthday. We had a party for him at the home. It was the most people he had at one of his birthday parties in a long time! We had cake and coffee and he got a lot of cards. I got a quilt for his bed and Heather brought cookies from our favorite bakery. He really seemed to enjoy it.

Tonight I went for my walk along the same route as last night and met no one! While there was no caring compassion, I also did not have to recount my trials and tribulations to anyone. The solitude was nice.

August 10, 2000

When Jack went into the nursing home, I gave him a blank journal. On the first page I wrote, "To Jack- I love you! Rose." A few days later he showed the journal to me. On the second page he had written, "To Rose. This is Jack. I love you too!" Today he showed it to me again. He pointed to my name and said, "I hope she stops by some day soon." I told him that I was Rose. He said, "Really? What is your last name?" I said, "I am Rose Grant. I am your wife." He seemed pleasantly surprised and said. "Well! We're going to have a lot more fun tonight than I thought!"

January, 2001

(NOTE: This entry is being written from memory as I couldn't write at the time it occurred.)

One day while I was at school, I got a call from a social worker at the nursing home. It seems that Jack had been getting harder and harder to handle, being resistant to daily care and combative during the night. He is a big man (6 feet tall and 170 lbs) and although his mind is weak, his body is still strong.

There had been some incidents of shoving and even hitting the staff. They had tried to control his behavior by readjusting his medications, but this wasn't working. They wanted to send him out to a geriatric/psychiatric hospital for evaluation. I was really upset about this, but didn't see that I had a choice. As it turned out, due to our medical coverage and limited placement choices, he was sent to Norwood Hospital. This facility is an hour from our home and a bit longer from my workplace. The day he was moved, I was told that I had to be there when he was admitted, which meant taking time off from work. I drove there only to be told that I wasn't allowed in (they had specific visiting hours) and they were busy taking his medical history anyway (from HIM?! HA!). After about an hour wait, they buzzed me into the locked unit. It was as if I had stepped onto the set of *One Flew Over the Cuckoo's Nest*. The unit had all sorts of people, most not Alzheimer's, who were there because they were very mentally ill and needed to have medication adjustments just like Jack. I personally found it very frightening and was worried about how Jack was going to deal with being in a different place. As it turned out, he didn't even notice that he wasn't at Country Gardens, so there was no problem with that. I was told that he would be there for seven to ten days. I tried to make the trip up every day after work and spent two hours with him, leaving after I helped him with supper. But adding the time for the commute after working all day and not getting supper until 7:30 PM had started to take its toll. I told myself that is was only temporary when ten days stretched into two weeks and there was still no sign of release.

While walking through the business office at school one morning at break time, I was told that I had a phone call. The woman on the other end informed me that she was a lawyer who had been appointed to represent my husband, who was about "to lose his liberty." I was trembling and could barely keep what she was saying straight. Evidently because he was involuntarily admitted to a psychiatric hospital, they had the right to send him to a more permanent placement rather than return him to the nursing home. She had been appointed as his public defender, so to speak. I was flabbergasted! She demanded a long list of documents she needed to prepare for court, which I had at home. After frantic calls to our own lawyer, the nursing home and others, I got my classes covered and went home to gather these papers. This lawyer was going to meet me at the nursing home to get the papers as well as look at Jack's records there. In the mean time, we got the lawyers for the hospital on the phone and discovered that it had been over looked that I was his health care proxy and could give permission for his care. This whole incident was the result of a misunderstanding and an overzealous lawyer. I drove to the hospital in Norwood and signed papers, giving them permission to extend Jack's stay. It was a nightmare!

Finally, about two and one half weeks later, he came back to the nursing home and seemed to be better.

February 26, 2001

A few days ago I was visiting Jack and he was talking away. Most of it was gibberish, so I asked him what language he was speaking and, without missing a beat, he said "Vesmeldick!" The universal language of Alzheimer's, I guess.

Jack doesn't remember to wash his hands after using the toilet, so if I am there I try to get him to do so. Most of the time, he doesn't know what I want him to do, so I get him in front of the sink and wash my hands and he will copy me (this is a technique called modeling). Last week even that didn't work, so I pulled his hands into the stream of water and handed him the bar of soap, which he promptly bit! At least his teeth were clean! Later on the same visit we both sat down to have an orange. I peeled his, sectioned it and put it on a napkin in front of him. His appetite is still excellent and he really seemed to enjoy the orange (it probably tasted quite good after the soap!). After the last bite, he began ripping up the napkin and stuck a long section of that in his mouth. I quickly retrieved that and disposed of the rest of it. They say that AD patients regress back in time. The incidents of this visit and the fact that Jack is now permanently in briefs (adult diapers) made me realize how much he now has in common with our eleven month old granddaughter. She loves to eat paper, too.

March 1, 2001

As a high school teacher, you would think I would be able to handle 16 elderly people in a nursing home dining room when I can handle lunch duty with 400 teenagers in attendance. Each night I help serve the supper trays to the residents who are still able to feed themselves. This gives me an easy way to separate myself from Jack at the end of the visit because he gets so engrossed in his food that he does not notice when I leave.

While they wait for the food truck to come down from the kitchen, the activities person often plays games such as Name That Tune, Proverbs (a type of word association) or Trivia. Often the answers given are much funnier than the correct ones, such as:

> "What can we find on the top of a television set and
> a bunny's head?" (those readers of the cable TV era
> might not get this!)
> ANSWER: "Dust!"

> "You can't see the forest for the…"
> ANSWER: "Forest fire!"

> "You can't get blood from a …"
> ANSWER: "Pumpkin!"

Tonight the answers were particularly hilarious and we were all laughing and having so much fun with it when, finally, the food arrived. Most of the funny answers came from this tiny, distinguished lady sitting next to my husband. But her personality took an about face when I placed her supper of grilled cheese and clam chowder in front of her. She started yelling that she didn't want that black stuff (the sandwich). Take it away! I did so, moving the bowl of chowder in its place. Her complaints escalated and got louder and the next thing I knew, she was reaching for her neighbor's chowder. With a bowl of hot chowder in each hand, she was about to fling them across the room just as I grabbed them. She immediately hauled off and punched me! She then assaulted me with a barrage of expletives just as the nurses arrived to escort her from the room. What a feisty 95 year old!

I was not hurt and understand the behavior of a typical AD resident. The activities aide told me later that she could almost see it coming. This resident almost always has a catastrophic episode after she is particularly amusing. What a strange disease this is.

June 23, 2001

Gus died last night. That makes four of the original six men at Country Gardens who are gone: Ed, Frank, Ray and now Gus. Only Jack and his roommate, Hank, are still with us. I passed by Gus' room and saw the aides packing up his things. One of the girls had his cap on her head and my first reaction was that she was making fun of him. The other girl said "Are you going to keep that?" and she replied, "Yes, I want a memento." I was really touched by that. I only got to know this man for the last 15 months of his life and what I saw was a grumpy, slow old man who did not talk much and who spat on the floor all the time. This young lady had been his aide all of the time he was a resident and she obviously had a very different memory of him. As she finished her shift, we walked out to the parking lot together. She was wearing Gus' cap and clutching a picture of him. I hope when it is Jack's turn that the staff will miss him as much.

July 6, 2001

Heather and I just returned from a ten-day trip to the Pacific Northwest. It was my graduation present to her. We spent three days in Seattle, Washington, three in Vancouver, Canada, and three in the Olympic National Park area. It was the longest I have ever been away from Jack in twenty-eight years of marriage. When I went to see him on the Fourth of July, I thought, "This is it. He definitely won't remember me now." I was tense and close to crying as I got to the nursing home and as I approached him, he ignored me. I planted myself right in front of him and gave him a hug. He looked at me and said, "Hello, love! I really have missed you." It made my day.

CHAPTER EIGHT

Stage III

———————

January 23, 2002

People are always asking me if Jack still recognizes me when I visit him. Most of the time now he does not. Sometimes I will walk right up to him when I arrive at the nursing home and say hello, and he will side-step me and not even acknowledge a person in front of him. Other times he will take me by both elbows and shove me aside as though I was a chair that he needs to push out of the way.

Yesterday, however, I found him sitting in a chair and greeted him by taking both of his hands in mine. He picked up each of my hands individually and kissed the backs of them. It was a very special moment for me. A few weeks ago I visited with our 20-month old granddaughter Meaghan. When he saw both of us he said, "Here's my peachy girls!" I live for these brief times when the little lucid windows in his brain open up.

January 24, 2002

I have suddenly become an "expert" on Alzheimer's disease and nursing homes. I would rather not know anything about either of these subjects, but here I am. In the past week, I have been on the phone for hours with people looking for advice about how to handle their loved one with AD or how to go about placing them in a facility. I don't mind helping people because so many people have helped me: I just hope I am giving good advice.

January 30, 2002

I went to visit Jack yesterday and found him on the floor in his room. He was wedged between the bed and his night stand and there was blood near him. His body was twitching from head to toe. I ran to the nurse's station for help and everyone came running. They assessed the situation and got him up in a wheelchair. After checking his vitals, they cleaned the cut on his hand (thus the blood on the floor). He didn't seem quite right to me, but he was alert and the twitching eventually subsided. Supper arrived and the nurses suggested that I try giving him some soup. This was not working very well, as the broth was just dribbling from his mouth. He also kept trying to lift his left arm, but it was very floppy. I pointed out both things to the nurses and said that it seemed to me that he might have had a stroke. We all agreed that he should go to the hospital and the necessary phone calls were made. He was transported to the hospital in Fall River by ambulance and I met him there.

The waiting room was standing room only and the triage nurse told me the wait was up to four hours long. Since Jack had been brought in by ambulance, we would be seen sooner and they brought me in back about an hour later. By this time they had done some tests-vitals, blood work, EKG. They had him on oxygen and hooked up to a monitor. I was a wreak and he was sound asleep! Sometime later, they took him for a CAT scan of his head and X-rays of his chest in case he had broken any ribs in the fall. At this point it was about 9 PM and I had not had dinner. They told me they were going to admit him, so I used his absence to make some phone calls, including calling in sick for work the next day, and to get something to eat.

When I got back, he was being wheeled back into the ER. After another wait, the doctor came in and said all of his tests came back normal. He said Jack could have had a seizure and that was why he was sleeping so soundly. The CAT scan showed no signs of a stroke. Since it was 11 PM, the doctor suggested that I go home to sleep. The hospital was nearly full and they were going to have to wait for a bed for him anyway.

I drove the five minute ride home. Let the cat in and picked up the mail. Five minutes later the phone rang. The ER doctor was on the phone telling me to get right back there as all of Jack's vital signs were falling rapidly. I was stunned. He said to "gather up the family because he probably won't make it through the night." I was trembling. I tried to reach our son, but he was still at work. Our daughter was in Kentucky, so there was no point in calling her. I called my brother-in-law Brian and then raced to the hospital.

The doctor told me it looked like a brain stem stroke, which doesn't often show up on a CAT scan, but is almost always cat-astrophic. I looked at him sleeping so peacefully and thought that this would be such a nice way for him to die. Brian and Shirley arrived. I filled them in and we began our bedside vigil. After a while I sent them home and at 2 AM they finally got a bed for him. I went upstairs with him and the nurses got him settled. They were very kind to me and explained that they would not put him on a monitor because there was no point and it was upsetting to watch his decline. This was true, as I was glued to it in the ER. They got a cot set up for me and it was at this point that I realized I was still in my sweaty aerobics clothes from my after school class the day before. Needless to say, I did not sleep much.

Early today, I went home and showered, changed clothes, took care of the cat, got coffee and came back to the hospital. I called my sister Carol, a nurse, about 6 AM and she came to the hospital to be with me. Brian also came in and the three of us sat there watching Jack sleep. I requested a priest who came in and anointed Jack. During the night on the cot I had been planning Jack's funeral, trying to decide what to do about Heather and when to call her. She cannot get here in time, especially if he died today, but I will need to call her in any case to let her know what is going on. Brian called Jack's mother and brothers and both David and Bill called the hospital room this morning.

About 10 AM a group of CNA trainees and their instructor came in and asked permission to reposition Jack in bed. I said yes and the three of us left the room. While we were in the hall, someone came down and said that Jack was very wet, so they were going to change him and the bed, and they would be a bit longer. This was fine with me. Finally, they let us back in the room and shortly after that Jack sat up in bed and started talking! Startled, I asked Carol how this could be possible and she said she didn't know. She said sometimes patients have these little rallies and then they die. She was warning me not to get my hopes up. But as the morning progressed he got more alert and more talkative. We put the back of the bed up and he tugged and twisted on the blanket all morning. His speech was clear but what he said made no sense and he was just blabbering to himself.

We waited all morning for the doctor to come and he finally arrived about 12:30 PM. It was the doctor covering for his own doctor, so I had never met him before. He said he was not expecting to see Jack sitting up talking; rather he expected to see a comatose patient. Now we were questioning whether he had a stroke or a grand mal seizure. Since no one had really seen what had happened to him and all of his tests were incon-clusive, we really had no way of knowing. He said he could have had an aborted stroke or a small blood clot that disintegrated. He suggested that Jack be evaluated by a neurologist and I agreed.

At this point, Jack had not had anything to eat or drink for almost 24 hours, so they started him on thickened liquids and later today he had several cups of pudding. He gobbled everything down. At about 9:30 PM tonight the neurologist came in, asked me a lot of questions, examined Jack and said he was leaning more toward a seizure. He suggested an EEG for the next day. Since Jack was so alert and this was not a secure unit, I decided to spend another night at the hospital.

January 31, 2002

Early this morning, I ran home for a shower and a change of clothes while Jack slept. He had his liquid breakfast and was taken for his brain wave. The technician was a former student of mine and was very kind to Jack. She explained the procedure to me, and as it went on, I tried to get information from her, but she was very professional and did not cooperate. A short time after Jack was brought back to his room, he was discharged and the ambulance arrived to take him back to the nursing home. Everyone back at Country Gardens was happy to see him (I had been calling them with updates from the ER and his room, so they too thought he was going to die). He was really enjoying the TLC and attention. After we got him settled, I came home.

Tonight I am exhausted and wracked with guilt. When I was told that Jack was going to die, it was upsetting but such a relief. I was so happy that he was going to die in his sleep and would never get to Stage III AD. He would not enter a vegetative state, being spoon fed mush. The kids and I would not have to remember him this way. Selfishly, I was also welcoming the end of Alzheimer's disease for me. I am at once happy to have my husband and disappointed that he did not die.

But, it is not yet time for Jack to go and I just have to trust God that He knows what He is doing.

February, 2002

Jack is now confined to a chair since the incident in January. He can walk with assistance and at times walks really well on his own, but for his own safety, he is in a geri-chair all day. Another loss. When he first came back from the hospital he was really sleepy all of the time and leaned over on his left side. His left arm also seemed to be weak. The hospital had sent him back with a stroke diagnosis, so all of this seemed to fit.

Since Jack is now immobile, he needs less medication and a pleasant side effect has been that he is much more alert and talkative. He will have great conversations with himself and laugh and laugh at what he says (only he gets this!). But we are all happy watching him have such a good time amusing himself and us in turn. It is almost as if a little of the old Jack is back.

Summer, 2002

For several months now Jack has been on a plateau. He is chair-bound, unable to communicate very much verbally and needs a great deal of assistance to eat. Since he is not ambulatory any more, he has put on a great deal of weight. His face is round and he has a big pot belly. When he entered Country Gardens, he barely weighed 150 pounds, mostly due to his constant walking and radiation treatment for cancer. He is now around 200 pounds.

The nursing home ordered a beautiful, high-backed wheel chair for him. Between his size and his strength, he was tipping a regular wheel chair over with no trouble at all. He gets himself all over the unit in this chair using foot power.

I managed to take two trips this summer. In July I went to Vermont with Heather for six days. We did some hiking, shopping, reading and relaxing. At the end of July, we drove to Louisville, Kentucky so that Heather could return to her apartment and job. From there, I flew to New Orleans, met up with my sister Pat and brother-in-law Ken and finished the week in Pensacola, Florida. While at Pat's, the home called to say that Jack had had a fall, but all in all it had been a pretty uneventful summer.

On August 12, the phone rang and woke me from a deep sleep. I missed the call and looked at the clock to discover it was 6:20 AM. I knew it had to be about Jack, so I called. He had just had a grand mal seizure and they wanted to know if I wanted him to go to the hospital. They had him in bed on oxygen and he seemed fine otherwise. I got right over there and he slept for five hours while I was there. By lunch he was up and eating, so all seems fine. They started him on anti-seizure medication and that seems to be helping. It makes me think now that what happened to him in January was also a seizure. I guess this is just one more indication of brain damage.

January, 2005

As of this writing, Jack has been in the nursing home almost five years. It is hard to believe this much time has gone by and that he is still alive. He is totally confined to a wheel chair and has been for some time. He has been incontinent for years now and rarely talks. Most of the time it is gibberish, but occasionally he will look right at you and say, "Hello" with a big smile on his face. He has to be fed pureed food and in recent months was "demoted" to having his liquids thickened to pudding consistency. He was having trouble swallowing.

Three years ago, Jack had his first event where he had a massive seizure, was pronounced at death's door and anointed by a priest, only to recover. He has since done this three more times, to different degrees. One time he appeared to be comatose for weeks, with very low vital signs, little intake of food or water and no response to stimuli. Hospice came in to take over his care and little by little he got better. He actually became a Hospice dropout! The most recent episode was just a couple of weeks ago. When this first happened, I sat praying for him and planning his funeral. Once I even bought the black dress. Now, I just play the waiting game and so far he has decided to stay on this planet. It is out of our hands.

January, 2006

As the year of 2005 progressed, so did Jack's deterioration. He could no longer do anything for himself. Small, but constant, seizures continued to wrack his body and his inability to swallow became more and more apparent. Yet he still hung in there. He developed pneumonia and skin issues but his heart was strong and he put up a good fight. Finally, around Christmas, he stopped swallowing almost completely. This made it difficult not only to get food into him but his medications as well. Without them, his seizures got worse. At times his body was almost constantly jerking in his bed. Because we had both drawn up advanced directives many years ago, I knew that he did not want artificial hydration or feeding, so we instituted comfort care only. He was given pain medication by suppository and placed on oxygen. On January 7th he began showing signs that the end was coming. Our children and their significant others were at his bedside. All of my family as well as Jack's brother and sister-in-law came by. During the day, a friend from school came and prayed the Chaplet of Divine Mercy for him. The kids and I stayed until about 3 AM and then all of us came home to sleep. I slept on the couch, fully clothed, with the phone beside me and at 6:30 AM the call came to hurry back. I got to Jack's room, kissed him and held his hand and he died a few minutes later. It was the peaceful death we were all praying for. I am grateful that I was able to be there with him when he finally left this world and all of the suffering he had endured for all those years.

CHAPTER NINE

Life After Alzheimer's

Jack was buried on a cold January day in St. Patrick's Cemetery, alongside his mom and dad. As a former Marine, he received military honors and the ceremony was very moving.

When our daughter Heather was born in January, of 1979, Jack sent an arrangement of roses and heather to the hospital. I was so surprised that he thought of that combination of flowers and he told me they had a hard time getting heather at that time of year. So, of course, I ordered the same two flowers for his casket arrangement and it was beautiful. We received many other flowers and they looked so lovely in the snow on his grave.

The day after his funeral, my children returned to their homes and I went back to work. I wanted to get my life back in order as soon as possible and the best place for me to be was with my colleagues and my students. Right after school, I drove to the cemetery to visit with Jack. I had heard that people will come after funerals to steal flowers and when I got to Jack's grave, I noticed that most of the roses were gone, the chrysanthemums were all pulled apart and in general the grave was a mess! I started crying at the cruelty of some thoughtless people when I saw deer tracks all around in the snow. My tears quickly turned to laughter when I realized I had spent $400 for deer food! Jack would have loved sharing his flowers with these beautiful creatures.

As time passed, each day got easier. It was an adjustment not to have to go to the nursing home every day, to not be a caregiver anymore, after twelve long years, and I thought I was doing fine. Every now and then the finality of it would sneak up on me and I would start crying. Sometimes I would have to pull the car over to the side of the road because I was sobbing so hard. As the months passed, my crying bouts happened less and less. My family and friends were loving and supportive and I started to heal. Someone who had traveled this rocky road before me advised me to "turn your grief into action." I decided to give it a try.

I got back to dedicating myself to being a good teacher and an organized prom planner. I got my much neglected house in order, cleaning and painting and redecorating. I gave myself a "new" bedroom, painted a very girly "Wisteria". I culled Jack's books and sold many to a good friend for his used book store. My kids claimed some of his clothes and the rest went to the Salvation Army.

Just as my house was neglected, so was my body. I had not had a real checkup in years, so I scheduled dental and doctor appointments. I was appalled to discover that my weight had climbed to 170 pounds (on my slightly over 5 foot frame)! My blood work numbers reflected my sorry state, so I joined Weight Watchers and lost almost 40 pounds. It took a while but my cholesterol came down an equal number of points, my joints no longer hurt and I dropped four sizes in clothes.

Now if I could only heal my lonely heart. I tried going to the movies and restaurants alone, but these trips only made my singleness more evident. My friends would invite me out with them, but I was the stag with all of the couples. When everyone got up to dance, I was left alone at the table. I started turning down their invitations. I tried on-line dating, which was a disaster. I hated trying to "sell" myself to strangers.

Then one day I got a call from an old high school friend. He asked to meet for coffee. We did and talked for three hours. We started visiting whenever he was in town and I finally had someone to cook for and eat with again, someone to walk with and laugh with and just be with. Many years later he is still my traveling companion, my confident and my best friend. Jack will never be replaced, but I am no longer lonely.

In the meantime, I have had wonderful groups of enthusiastic students walk with me as members of my "Jack's Pack" team in the Walk to End Alzheimer's. With their help, we have raised awareness and funds for research totaling over $100,000. I have become a certified bioethicist and a support group co-facilitator. I lecture and sit on panels for Alzheimer's caregiving and education. I am an active member of the Southeastern Massachusetts Alzheimer's Partnership.

In the spring of 2014, I was fortunate to have a story about Jack published in *Chicken Soup for the Soul-Living with Alzheimer's and other Dementias.* This kept me occupied for some time with readings and book signings at such places as the Massachusetts State House and Patriot's Place. It was exciting to raise awareness and money for my team and the Alzheimer's Association in this way.

After thirty-eight years in the classroom, I retired from teaching in June of 2013. I now have time to devote to my passions: gardening, quilting, traveling and the one passion I did not choose: Alzheimer's disease. I co-facilitate a support group for early on-set AD couples, I lecture at the local university in gerontology and nursing classes, and I work tirelessly to educate others about this terrible disease that came into my life uninvited. I annually make over sixty jars of jam and jelly for my "Jammin for Jack" fundraiser for my team and each year I organize a "Summer Memories" party to continue to raise funds for research, support and education. "Turn your grief into action" has become my motto.

Life is good again. I am happy, healthy and fulfilled. I have found ways to honor Jack's memory and to try to pay it forward, to thank all of those who have helped me along the way. I hope in some small way this bittersweet story of our journey will help others living this "long goodbye."

Caregiver Help Notes

Chore Sheet

(This is a sample of a sheet that was left on a clip board by the phone for Jack. I re-did it every night for the next day.)

Today is: _____

(day of week and date)

Suggestions for things to do today:

_____Cut the grass

_____Make our bed

_____Empty the dishwasher

_____Feed the cat

_____Take a walk

Suggestions for lunch:

_____Homemade chicken soup

_____Tuna salad sandwich

_____Bagel with cream cheese

I will be home by 3 PM. We have a doctor's appointment at 4 PM.

If you need me call Bishop Stang at 508-555-1234.

Love you! Rose

Hospitalization of an Alzheimer's Patient

You need to realize that there are medical personnel who are ignorant about Alzheimer's disease. I have encountered many nurses and doctors who seem to know very little about the symptoms and behaviors of someone with this type of dementia. When Jack went for his colonoscopy (bowel study), the nurse did not want me to accompany him when he was being prepped for the procedure. Even though I had informed her that he had AD, she told me that "there are tight quarters back there." As she prepared Jack and began to take a medical history from him, she realized why I needed to be there. His answer to why he was having a colonoscopy was because his memory was bad!

We are all frightened when we go to the hospital. After all, we are there because we are very sick, have been in an accident or need surgery. Imagine how scary the hospital must be to an Alzheimer's patient. Nothing and no one is familiar. Strangers are doing things to you and many of those things hurt. Hospitals are also places of stimulation overload. There are lots of people, lots of noises (even in the middle of the night), unfamiliar smells and all kinds of pokes and prods.

Here are some suggestions to make things easier for you and your family member:

- Although most hospitals now have private rooms, some do not. Try to get a private room if your medical insurance will cover it. Sometimes it takes a doctor's order and it may not occur to her until you ask.

- Unless your family member is addicted to television, I would leave it off. There are too many other sources of noise in the hospital to distract and upset the patient. Instead, I brought a small radio from home and played classical music softly in the background. That seemed to quiet Jack.

• Bring other items from home that may make the patient think he is home- a favorite bathrobe or sweater, pillow, photos of family, or flowers from your garden.

• Dim the lights whenever possible.

• Minimize the visitors and phone calls. Perhaps relatives can take shifts to allow others to go home. Use this time for yourself: a nap, shower, a good meal, a walk with the dog.

• If your doctor will order someone to sit with the patient overnight or when you can't be there, take advantage of this. Again, you might have to look at whether insurance will pay for this. Don't wait for this to be suggested. You might have to take the initiative (see #1).

• Make sure directions to the patient are clear and brief. Be sure the person giving them is making eye contact and has the patient's attention. Only tell the patient what he really needs to know. Give the details to the family member. (I once had a lab tech give Jack detailed directions for a clean catch urine specimen. It was almost laughable that she would expect him to be able to accomplish this.)

• Too many people interacting with the patient may be overwhelming. See if the hospital is willing to assign specific people to your family member while they are there. This may not be practical or possible but it is worth a try.

• Consult with a psychiatrist or Alzheimer's specialist on the hospital staff to be sure the medication the patient is receiving is appropriate and will not aggravate the confusion and agitation.

Letter to Volunteer Day Care Help

August 25, 1999

Dear Friends of Jack Grant:

As you know, Jack has been diagnosed with Alzheimer's disease (AD). So far, he is holding his own and is doing well, all things considered. His major issues right now are short-term memory and language problems, including both coming up with words he wants and understanding things spoken to him.

I am going back to school next week and am anxious about leaving him alone all day. This worked fine last year but I have seen signs this summer that we might not be able to continue with this through this school year. Both Jack and I feel very strongly about keeping him home for as long as possible. That is why I am writing to you.

Rather than put Jack into adult day care or having strangers take care of him, I am hoping that enough of you would be able and interested in spending one day a week with Jack in our home so that he can stay here while I am at work. I would be able to pay you around $30 a day plus lunch. While this is not much, it would be cash and maybe some extra pocket money for you.

Here's what I anticipate as a typical day:

> Arrive at our house between 7:00 and 7:15 AM-
> Rose leaves for work
> Assist/supervise Jack's household chores/yard work
> Coffee break- Jack likes to go for coffee/muffin each
> morning around 10:00 AM
> Go for a walk or walk to the coffee break location
> Reading time
> Lunch

Errands/another walk/reading
Rose home by 3:00 PM

Right now Jack goes to the Boys' Club three mornings a week-Monday, Wednesday and Friday. If you came on one of those days, that would take up a good part of the morning. Obviously, this schedule is flexible. If you had errands to do, he could certainly go along for the ride so you could probably get some of your own things done. Things do go best for Jack, however, when a routine is maintained.

Jack does not know that I am writing this letter to you, although we have discussed this plan I am currently suggesting to you and he was happy about it. I am asking you to respond by filling out the form below and sending it to me in the enclosed envelope. I realize that some of you have more time available than others but I need to plan ahead and have some idea if this is workable. Think about it and let me know if you are interested.

Thanks so much!

Rose

Response: (check one)

_____I would love to help, but my schedule is already quite full! I will keep Jack in my thoughts and prayers.

_____The money and free lunch sound great! How can I turn them down? Please call me.

_____I need more time/information before I can make a commitment. Please call me when the plan is going to be put into action.

Your Name: _____

Phone: _____

Day Care Schedule: Jack's Companions

Week of: _____

Monday 7 am-11 am	Tuesday	Wednesday	Thursday	Friday
11 am-3 pm				

NAMES: PHONE:

Don ----

Brian ----

Bill -----

Kevin -----

Charlene -----

Carol -----

Jim-----

Bathrooms

Public

We need to advocate for more unisex/family bathrooms in public places. Many malls now have them but they are still few and far between. Many parents have already faced this issue-what does Dad do when he is out alone with his 4 year old daughter who needs to "potty?" This is really the same issue for Alzheimer's Disease- the child is just in the adult's body. While your patient is still somewhat aware (Stage I or II AD), you also want to avoid embarrassing him. I have discreetly asked for a gentleman's help for Jack and most people are good. But once a man just yelled and yelled at him because he couldn't understand the lock on the bathroom door and I ended up IN THE MENS' ROOM! We do what we have to do.

At Home

Many AD patients obsess about the bathroom. At times Jack was going to the bathroom every fifteen minutes. He would often use the bathroom downstairs, come out and go right upstairs to use the other one.

During the night finding the bathroom became a real issue for Jack as well as finding his way back to bed. I got large signs (8" x 10") that said "toilet" with a picture of toilet and another that said "Jack's room" with a picture of a bed and posted these on the appropriate doors. These are also very helpful to take when traveling. You might want to have them laminated. Jack hated my sister's beautiful house in Maine because it had "too many doors." In hindsight, we now know why he disliked this house so much.

Legal Issues

If you can afford it (find a way!), hire a lawyer, particularly one who specializes in elder issues such as long term care and Medicare/Medicaid. Your local bar association and the Alzheimer's Association can give you a list of these individuals. You need to be sure to change legal documents that name your spouse as your beneficiary or health care proxy, for example. The lawyer will know what you need to do and what kind of documentation you will need to provide. We qualified for Medicaid, but that meant providing three years' worth of bank statements, utility bills, insurance, tax returns- a mound of paperwork. Remember you will be doing this while trying to take care of an AD patient and possibly working as I was. You are also stressed with the idea that you are placing your loved one in a nursing home. This is a great time to get help and well worth the expense.

Although most states will no longer make a spouse sell their home to help pay for care, we did put the house in my name only as soon as Jack was diagnosed in 1995. Do not procrastinate about taking care of legal issues. If you do some of this while your relative is in the early stages, he will be able to participate and have his wishes known and carried out. Also, now is the time to get records and paper work in order. I had all of our bank statements, but they were haphazardly "filed" in a shoebox in the basement in no order. Now I have large binders that they go in as I receive them. This makes my life so much easier in case someone requests them. If the AD patient is your parent or an elderly relative, this is even more imperative since you may not know where these papers are at all.

Another piece of advice: photocopy EVERYTHING before you send it out. I was asked for the same document several times. I would have been in trouble had I not kept copies. Many times you are given deadlines by Medicaid that do not give you a great deal of time to provide that paperwork (one December I received a re-determination for eligibility for Medicaid form on December 20 and it was due in their office on December 24. This was the weekend before Christmas! The nursing home social worker called the field office and asked for an extension, but I was denied. The moral of this story is to be ready!)

Identification Bracelets

My husband Jack was a great walker and this did not change when he got Alzheimer's. From his journal, you read that walking each day was an important part of his life, but as time progressed I worried more and more about him finding his way home. Incidents like getting lost on the beach and jumping out of our car really scared me. Over half of dementia patients will wander and most who do are repeat offenders. We can't always count on our loved one having identification on them or remembering their address or phone number. Here are a couple of options:

Medic Alert and the Alzheimer's Association have teamed up to provide a 24-hour national emergency program called Safe Return. For an initial fee, the patient is given an identification bracelet to wear. It indicates memory impairment and has an 800 number on the bracelet to call if the person is found wandering or lost. There is also a specific ID number assigned to your loved one and this will help to identify him, give emergency contacts, list his medications and even allows a photograph to be on file. If a person wearing the bracelet is reported missing, a search and rescue is then initiated. A smaller renewal fee is charged and an opportunity to update information occurs annually. The clasp on this bracelet is very hard to manipulate and the family member cannot remove it on their own. (1-800-572-8566)

An alternative is the Project Life Saver bracelet, issued by your sheriff's department. This bracelet is attached to the wrist of your loved one by a member of your local sheriff's office. It looks somewhat like a watch and can be worn while swimming or bathing. It must be cut off to be removed and the battery must be changed by sheriff department personnel once a month. The bracelet emits a radio frequency signal, specifically assigned to the individual, which helps to locate the person if she goes missing.

There are pros and cons to each bracelet. Safe Return is much cheaper than the Project Life Saver bracelet (the initial cost is several hundred dollars) but it does not have electronic monitoring capabilities. The radio signal, however, only has a range of about 1 mile, so if your family member got on a bus and traveled far from home, the system would not work. Some people object to having a law enforcement person come to their house once a month to change the battery. Somehow this feels wrong to them. "Mom is not a criminal on house confinement." We have to remember that we are trying to keep our family member safe.

It might be a good idea for the caregiver to also wear a bracelet. Medic Alert has one for this purpose. Our local Alzheimer's Partnership has designed and distributes a caregiver bracelet, accompanied by a card stating who they care for, where this person resides, and who their backup contacts are. This was initiated when we heard about a caregiver who left his wife at home while he made a brief trip to the post office. While there, he had a stroke and was rushed to the hospital. He could not talk and his wife was left at home alone for hours, with no meds and no food.

One last thought on this. Let your local police department know of your situation and have an up to date photograph of your family member ready in case you need it. Hopefully, you will never have to use it, but better safe than sorry.

Eating Out

Depending on the stage that your family member is in, you will have to decide if he or she can handle going to a restaurant. Sometimes the change in routine and the commotion (noise, so many other people) are too upsetting. Trying to figure out a menu may be overwhelming to the AD person. If you really want to eat out and they like to, too, you might make things easier by going to a favorite place where you are known. You may want to call ahead and let them know of your situation, especially if they don't know you or the fact that someone in your party has Alzheimer's disease. Since Jack got too upset reading a menu and listening to the choices, I wish I had thought to also pre-order our meal. Instead of being presented with menus, I could have said, "Just bring us the usual!" During that incident where Jack's food was late, I wish I had just thought to give him my plate. He probably wouldn't have remembered what he ordered and we might have avoided upsetting him.

Many of the nursing home residents continue to go out with family members to eat, so I know they could handle it. I guess it is just an individual thing. What will upsct one person will be fine with another.

Post Office and Safety Deposit Boxes

All of Jack's income streams (three sources at the time) were sent to the bank via direct deposit but at least two of these sources sent us "dummy" pay stubs monthly or quarterly.

When the mail came while I was at work, Jack would see these stubs and get upset trying to understand them. Month after month I would go through the explanation. Initially, I wrote it all out, sat down and explained it and had Jack read, sign and date it. This was done because month after month he would claim that this was all new to him. Sometimes he would accuse me of stealing his money.

I finally got the idea to open a post office box for all first class mail. This allowed junk mail and magazines to still come to the house since Jack looked forward to getting the mail. My letter carriers were aware of Jack's situation and this gave me the opportunity of having a daily check on him while he was home alone.

One day I came home from school to find the contents of a cabinet spread out on the dining room floor. This was where I kept all of our important papers-the deed to the house, our passports, medical records, college diplomas and so on. Jack had these things all over the place. A grand day of rummaging! This prompted me to get a safety deposit box for any papers that I could not easily replace. It is really best to get these things out of the house because, at least in my case, Jack got into places he never would have in the past. His hiding places turned out to be very bizarre. My daughter found old photographs, face toward the wall, tucked into the molding inside her clothes closet! You might want to consider moving other valuables (grandma's crystal, your wedding pictures, and other family heirlooms) to someone else's house to avoid damage to them.

For less than $50 annually, these two boxes gave me some peace of mind.

Nursing Home Placement

While this was unique to my situation, I found myself doing a Medicaid application, federal and state tax returns, and college financial aid applications all at the same time. All of this was happening while working full time and taking care of Jack, with nursing home placement right around the corner. I did have a lawyer and accountant helping me, but the numbers and the records still had to come from me. It was overwhelming.

Since I was a rookie at nursing home placement, there was a lot I did not know and therefore did not ask the right questions at times. My best advice to you would be to ask the nursing home for a checklist of what needs to be done before your family member is placed. Get another checklist from your attorney for the necessary documentation you must supply.

Five years after I placed Jack in a nursing home, I was asked to participate in a panel discussion. I was so much smarter and wiser by then. What follows are some of my notes from that talk, plus the handout I created for that presentation.

How do you know when it is time for your family member to go into the nursing home?

- A nurse friend of mine (whose mother had AD) said, "Husbands place their wives in nursing homes too soon and wives place their husbands too late."

- Our doctor said," You will know it is time (to place your loved one in a nursing home) when YOU are not able to do your day job, when YOU are not getting enough sleep and when YOU are getting sick."

- Our daughter said, "Why are you trying so hard to keep Dad home when he doesn't know where home is anymore?"

All of these were reality checks for me. There are also many practical reasons for placement:

- Are there safety issues for your family member with AD and for those who live with him by keeping him at home?

- Is this person having more accidents? Is he leaving the stove on? Is he wandering and getting lost?

- Has the care of this family member at home become too much of a physical burden for the caregiver? Is the caregiver also elderly, frail or in poor health?

- Do you need to remodel or reconfigure your house to keep this person at home? Can you afford to do this?

Suggestions Before and During
the Placement Process-
Thoughts from Rose Grant, Family Member
Country Gardens Nursing Home

Swansea, MA   **November 30, 2005**

• **Get paperwork in order!!** Medical records, health care proxies, living wills, insurance cards, deeds, bank statements, burial plans, utility bills, income tax records, etc, etc, etc!! Not only will the nursing home need many of these, you will need them for the past three years if you are going to apply for Medicaid. If you are the primary caregiver, this may be an overwhelming job while you are also providing care. Try to do this well before you may need these documents.

• **Get help!** Go to a support group. Contact all of your friends (you'll at least find out who the real ones are). See if your church has a respite committee. Purchase *The 36 Hour Day- A Family Guide in Caring for a Person with Alzheimer's Disease* by Nancy L. Mace and Peter V. Rabins. Contact www. alzmass.org or your local Elder Services.

• **Get advice!** Talk to your doctors, to friends who have been there and done that, to social workers. The professionals may not agree with this, but avoid people who have no clue about Alzheimer's disease. Some of these well-meaning, but ill informed, individuals did me more harm than good. Hire a lawyer experienced in elder issues. It will be money well spent.

• **Get a feel for the lay of the land!** Visit facilities in your area to see what they have to offer. I was told not to be swayed by beautiful furniture and pretty pictures on the walls. Good advice! Ask yourself-is the facility clean? Does the staff interact with the residents in a loving and patient way? Are they trained in the care of AD residents? Bring a list with you of what is important to your loved one. Is he a religious individual who would want to go to mass? Is that available? Is your mother someone who was always well groomed? Do they have a salon or a hairdresser available? Do they have a safe outdoor place for enjoying a sunny day? Do they have music and activities that your family member would enjoy?

• **Get a checklist!** Once you decide on a facility and a placement time frame, ask the nursing home for a checklist of the things you need to do prior to placement. It is such an emotional time that you may not be thinking clearly.

• **Get it done!** Once you have made the difficult decision to place your family member in a nursing home, DO IT! Try not to agonize over your decision or beat yourself up over it. You are both going to be better cared for, safer and more at peace. You will finally have time for that doctor's appointment you have put off for three years. Once you realize that your family member is getting competent, professional, twenty-four hour care you might actually relax enough to go on a vacation and not feel guilty about it. You have actually just made the best, most thoughtful and loving decision you ever could have for this special person in your life. Give yourself a pat on the back for a job well done!

Visiting the Nursing Home

• One day at school, two of my friends and fellow teachers began giving me a hard time about the fact that I went to the nursing home almost every day. They were concerned about my health I'm sure, but my response was, "If this was your husband you would be there every day, too." They both insisted that they would not be there daily. I told them, "You two are either liars or bad wives!" We all laughed about it and went off to class.

Other people have asked why I bothered because Jack didn't know me any more or remember whether I had been. That is not the point. He may not have known me but I knew him. I needed to go for me. This is a very private and individual decision. When Jack was still at home, I had a 16-24 hour shift caring for him. When he was in the nursing home, I was down to an hour or so a day. I brought in his clean clothes, gathered up the dirty laundry and helped him with lunch or supper.

I did take days off and I did go on vacations. And I eventually got over feeling guilty about it. Visiting often and at different times allows you to see the place in action, to meet the staff, to see how they interact with the residents, to check on cleanliness, meals and so on.

• I brought a tote bag with me on each visit. In it I kept the following:

> Nail clippers
> Lotion
> Plastic bag for laundry
> Laundry pen
> Small sewing kit
> Pen & notebook
> Snacks
> Magazines/daily newspaper

You may want to adapt this to fit the interests of your family member-puzzles, music tapes or CDs, etc. As time goes on, their abilities will change and so will the contents of your bag.

• Clothing Issues

You know how your washing machine eats socks (but never two from the same pair)? Clothes seem to disappear at a regular rate in nursing homes. Some of it is a laundry issue, but most often it is just misplaced. Forget the stories about staff theft. Come on-who wants to steal some old lady's bra or old man's jockey shorts? One resident in my husband's home thought everything, including the building, belonged to her! When something was missing, they looked in her room first.

The number of missing items diminished as Jack settled into the routine of the home. His glasses were "hidden" in someone else's nightstand and I often found ladies glasses in his. Whether he did this or they did, who knows?

Obviously, everything should be labeled with the resident's name. I also kept a descriptive inventory of his clothes in the notebook in my tote bag. It helped to keep track of missing items and how often I replaced things.

Some people might not like this idea, but I bought Jack's clothing at discount and used clothing stores. I wanted him to be clean, comfortable and look nice. But it wasn't as upsetting if a $5 sweatshirt was missing versus a $40 sweater. Because his eating skills became so poor, he was staining his clothes a great deal, so expensive clothes were not practical.

Caregiving after Placement

Some people will be able to place their loved one in a nursing home, breathe a big sigh of relief, and let them take over. I personally think this is easier to do with a parent than a spouse, but in any case it was difficult for me to let go.

Jack was always very prudish. He never hung around the house in pajamas-much less in underwear! In his early days in the nursing home he was aware enough to realize that there was something wrong with being naked in front of a young woman he did not know who was trying to give him a shower. Since he was so resistant to care I knew I would get more cooperation and took it upon myself to do this job.

I also continued to do his laundry. He had always had problems with his skin and I could only use one brand of soap and detergent at home. Obviously, laundry done in a facility for many different people, most of whom are incontinent, must be done in very hot water with heavy duty detergent. Doing laundry at home treats it more kindly, prevents some clothing loss and, for me anyway, kept me connected to my husband. You may be glad to have one less thing to do.

Holiday Visits

Some of the residents in the nursing home were still really "with it" despite their memory problems, but Jack was not. He would not know that it was Christmas even if the tree was up and Santa was standing in front of him. So it did not make sense to make a big production out of the holidays for him. Of course, the production was important for the children and me. The first Christmas we all trouped in together with gaily decorated presents that we had put much thought into. He neither acknowledged them nor opened them. We had to open them for him and he still didn't pay any attention to them. It was just another day to Jack.

Country Gardens had dessert buffets for the families on all holidays. They were very nice but after the first couple we stopped going because Jack got too upset. The home was jammed with relatives who only visited on the major holidays, usually bringing lots of little children who ran around making lots of noise. This very big break in routine always got Jack agitated. What worked better for us was getting some desserts to have in the quiet of his room with just our immediate family.

Many families bring the family member home for the holiday for a day visit. You could see how she handles this. For Jack, I was afraid he would not want to go back and would be hard to handle. Obviously, you would have to weigh this for yourself. Really, most of the time, they do not know it is a holiday or whether they are at Aunt Margaret's, Stop & Shop or the nursing home. In this case, I would play it safe and keep the person where they are most comfortable.